Using This Book Is Simple

This book is designed for busy people. It is mainly graphic;
the drawings convey much of the information. Text is minimal.

HOW TO STRETCH

First read pages 4 to 7 for the basics on stretching.

GO BY THE FEEL

Next follow through the series of six stretches on pages 10 to 13. This
will teach you how to stretch.

STRETCHING ROUTINES

Skip ahead now and take a look at the routines on pages 19 to 39. They
are the heart of the book.

STRETCHING INSTRUCTIONS

Read the instructions for each of the stretches (*pp. 65 to 84*) the first
time you do them. (See the page reference under each stretch in the
routines.)

Then select a program and

S–T–R–E–T–C–H

STRETCHING
at your computer or desk

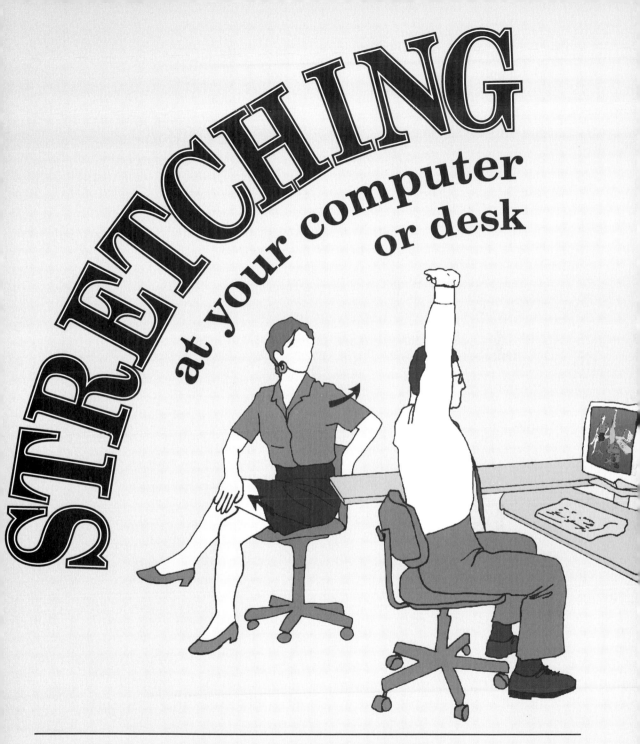

Bob Anderson
Illustrated by Jean Anderson

Distributed in the United States by Random House, Inc. and in Canada by Random House of Canada, Ltd., as agent for Shelter Publications, Inc.

Library of Congress Cataloging-in-Publication Data
Anderson, Bob, 1945–
    Stretching at your computer or desk / Bob Anderson; illustrated by Jean Anderson
        p.   cm.
    Includes bibliographical references and index.
    ISBN 0-936070-19-6 (Shelter) : $9.95.   ISBN 0-679-77084-4 (Random House)
    1. Stretching exercises.   2. Microcomputers—Health aspects.
3. Desks—Health aspects.   I. Anderson, Jean (Jean E.)   II. Title.
RA781.63.A53   1997
613.7'1—dc20   96-34996
                                                                                             CIP

We are grateful to Fellowes Computerware, Itasca, Illinois, for permission to reprint the drawing "Ergoman" on page 46.

7 6 5 4 3 2 1—03 02 01 00 99 98 97
(Lowest numbers indicate number and year of this printing)

Printed in the USA

This book has a RepKover® "lay-flat" binding. (Note how the spine is constructed.)

PLEASE NOTE: The stretches, exercises, and other information in this book are not meant to substitute for medical diagnosis and/or treatment. If you have any physical problems or health conditions, please consult with your physician or health professional before trying any new physical activity.

Write, call, or e-mail us for a free copy of our catalog:
Shelter Publications, Inc.
P.O. Box 279
Bolinas, CA 94924
415-868-0280
E-mail: shelter@shelterpub.com

VISIT US ON THE WEB: http://www.shelterpub.com

Other than the invention of the steam engine by Watt and the subsequent mechanization and industrialization of human work, perhaps no single technological advancement in how work is organized and performed has caused as much concern among humans, and their social and technical organizations, as the invention and subsequent proliferation of the computer.

Harry L. Davis, in foreword to
Ergonomics in Computerized Offices
Etienne Grandjean

Stretching

At Your Computer or Desk

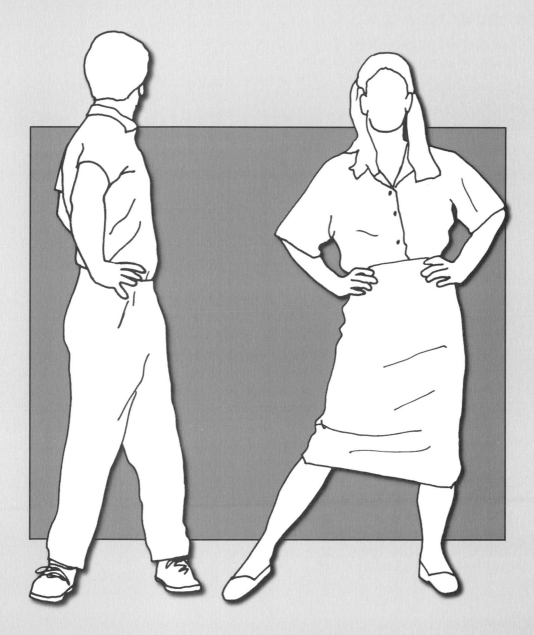

Contents

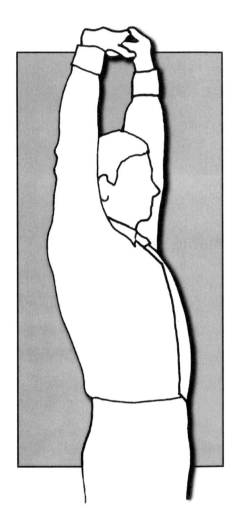

Contents

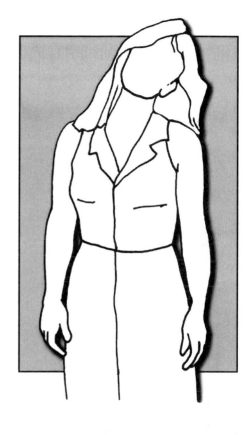

Introduction

A funny thing happened on the way to the electronic revolution. Large numbers of us ended up sitting at desks, working at computers. And that, as so many people have discovered, has its problems, its downsides.

Repetitive strain injuries (such as carpal tunnel syndrome and tendinitis) of the wrists, hands, and arms have risen by 80% since 1990, according to the U. S. Bureau of Labor Statistics, and are now the single largest category of workplace-related injuries. In fact, they are now being described as the workplace epidemic of the nineties.

Neck and shoulder stiffness, lower back pain, stiff muscles, and tight joints are all common among people working at computers. All of these conditions are the body signaling that something is wrong.

The human body was not designed for long periods of sitting. Holding still for hours at a time is a relatively recent phenomenon in human history. For some two million years, our ancestors had to use their bodies and muscles daily. In nomadic times activity was required for hunting and gathering. With the agricultural revolution, tilling the soil, planting, and harvesting required physical effort. After the industrial revolution and the advent of machines and motor vehicles, however, physical activity began to decline; nevertheless millions still worked in factories and assembly lines, using their bodies daily.

Now all that is changing — fast. The electronic revolution has meant that increasing numbers of people must spend more and more time sitting very still, working with computers, and the resultant problems are multiplying.

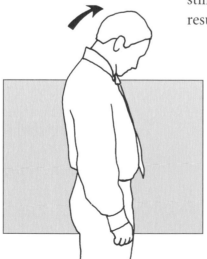

This book is for people who work at a computer and/or a desk and want to do something to counteract the negative effects that fixed positions and sedentary office work have on their bodies.

Stretching is a wonderful solution. It is a very simple activity that can make you feel better. It is gentle, peaceful, and relaxing. If practiced correctly, it can prevent many computer-related problems before they start and—if an injury has occurred—can help with rehabilitation.

Stretching can be done almost anywhere and at any time. It requires no special equipment, no special clothes, no special skills. You can stretch periodically throughout the day wherever you are. It can often be done while you are doing something else: when you're at an office meeting, while on the phone, or while you're waiting for the computer to process information.

Bob Anderson has taught stretching to people for almost 30 years and has seen gratifying results from this simplest of all physical activities — for people in all walks of life, from ordinary citizens to people in wheelchairs to world-class athletes.

This book applies the basic principles of stretching to the problems inherent in working at a computer and sitting still for long periods of time. It will show you how taking short stretching breaks throughout the day can make you feel better, prevent injuries, and lead to a more productive workday.

But first, let's take a closer look at typical problems of the computer workplace.

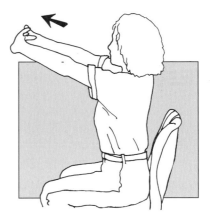

Computer & Desk Problems

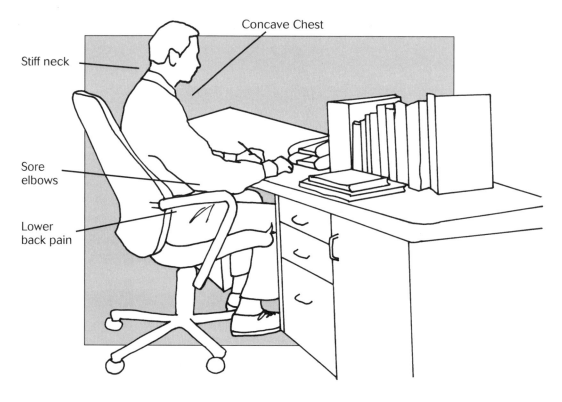

Stiff neck

Concave Chest

Sore elbows

Lower back pain

A typical desk setup

• **Back pain** When you sit for long periods, your spine tends to compress. If your posture is bad, gravity accentuates the problem, which can lead to back pain.

• **Stiff muscles** Not moving for long periods of time can cause neck and shoulder pain.

• **Tight joints** Inactivity can cause joints to tighten, which makes moving more difficult or even painful.

• **Poor circulation** When you sit very still, blood tends to settle in the lower legs and feet and does not circulate easily throughout the body.

• **Repetitive strain injuries** These injuries are caused by repetitive movement, often of the hands. For example, carpal tunnel syndrome, a type of wrist pain, can result from improper use of the hands and/ or poor positioning at the workstation.

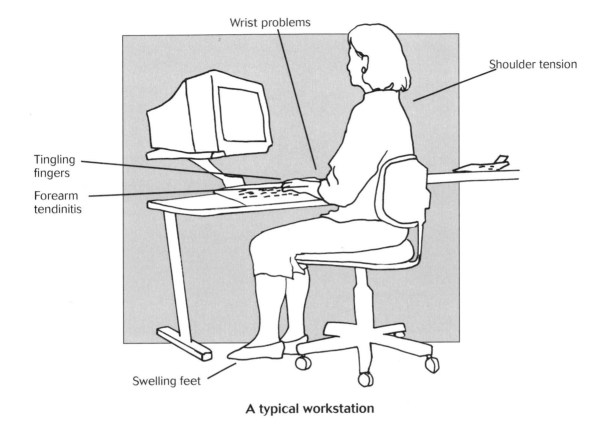

Wrist problems

Shoulder tension

Tingling fingers

Forearm tendinitis

Swelling feet

A typical workstation

• **Tension and stress** Intense mental focus can produce physical tension (stiffness and pain), which can lead to mental stress—a debilitating cycle. Facial tension and a tight jaw can cause headaches.

Many of these problems can be solved by ergonomics—the science involved with proper type and positioning of office equipment in relation to the body (*see pp. 46 to 50*). However, no matter how sound the ergonomics, your body still suffers from long periods of sitting and inactivity. What can you do throughout the long work day to help prevent these problems?

You can stretch!

When to Stretch

Stretching every hour or so throughout the day can help you avoid stiffness and muscle soreness, and make you feel better. You can stretch:

- On the job, to release nervous tension
- While your computer is processing something, if only for 5 to 10 seconds
- Whenever you feel stiff, sore, or tired
- Before and after taking a walk
- In the morning, just after getting up, and in the evening, before sleep
- When you need more energy
- Whenever you want to focus and do your best

Where to Stretch

You can stretch at your computer, or at your desk, and in a variety of other places. Here's a chance to be creative. For example, you can stretch:

- When you're a passenger in a car, or in a bus, or train on the way to work
- At your desk
- While on the phone
- At the copy machine
- At the filing cabinet or drinking fountain
- At office meetings
- While standing or waiting in line
- Before getting up to go anywhere

Benefits of Stretching

Stretching is just about the simplest of all physical activities. It is the perfect antidote for long periods of inactivity and holding still. Regular stretching throughout the day will:

- Reduce muscle tension
- Improve circulation
- Reduce anxiety, stress, and fatigue
- Improve mental alertness
- Decrease the risk of injury
- Make your work easier
- Tune your mind into your body
- Make you feel better!

IF YOU ARE INJURED

Please note: If you have an injury or any type of recurring soreness as described on pages 2 and 3, see a doctor or health care provider now. These stretches are not intended to cure serious problems. If you have the symptoms of a repetitive strain injury, some damage has already been done. If you do not take the right steps, damage could be permanent. For more details, see the section on repetitive strain injuries starting on page 44.

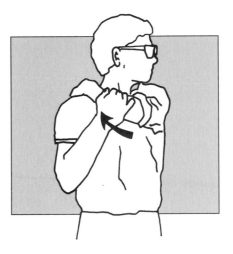

How to Stretch

THE RIGHT WAY TO STRETCH

- Breathe easily
- Relax
- Tune into your body
- Focus on muscles and joints being stretched
- *Feel* the stretch
- Be guided by the *feel* of the stretch
- No bouncing!
- No pain!

THE WRONG WAY TO STRETCH

- Holding your breath
- Being in a hurry
- Not being focused on your body
- Stretching while tense
- Bouncing
- Stretching to the point of pain

TWO PHASES

There are two phases to each stretch: the easy stretch and the developmental stretch. They are done one after the other.

THE EASY STRETCH

Stretch until you feel a slight mild tension and hold for 5–10 seconds. *Relax.* As you hold the stretch, the feeling of tension should diminish. If it doesn't, ease off slightly into a more comfortable stretch. The easy stretch maintains flexibility, loosens muscles and tight tendons, and reduces muscle tension.

THE DEVELOPMENTAL STRETCH

Now, move a fraction of an inch farther into the stretch until you feel mild tension again. Hold for 5 to 10 seconds. Again, the feeling should diminish or stay the same. If the tension increases or becomes painful, you are overstretching —back off into a more comfortable stretch. The developmental stretch further reduces tension and increases flexibility.

KEEP THE FOLLOWING POINTS IN MIND

- Always stretch within your comfortable limits, never to the point of pain.

- Breathe slowly, rhythmically and under control. Do not hold your breath.

- Take your time. The long-sustained, mild stretch reduces unwanted muscle tension and tightness.

- Do not compare yourself with others. We are all different. Comparisons may lead to overstretching.

- If you are stretching correctly, the stretch feeling should slightly subside as you hold the stretch.

- Any stretch that grows in intensity or becomes painful means you are overstretching—the drastic stretch. (See page 13.)

PAY ATTENTION TO HOW EACH STRETCH FEELS

Hold only stretch tensions that feel good. Relax while you concentrate on the area being stretched.

IMPORTANT

No bouncing
No pain

HOW FAR SHOULD I STRETCH?

Your body is different every day. Be guided by how the stretch feels.

STRETCHING IS NOT EXERCISE!

You are stretching, not exercising. You don't need to push it. Stretching is a mild, gentle activity.

GIVE IT 2 TO 3 WEEKS FOR BENEFITS

The benefits come from regularity. Stick with it and see how you feel in a few weeks.

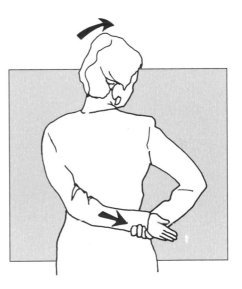

Watch a cat stretch. Cats are graceful and coordinated. They instinctively stretch to keep muscles tuned, joints flexible. Notice how the cat feels the stretch, tests the tension, relaxes, sometimes yawns, focuses on the stretch.

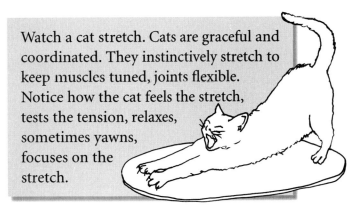

Go by the Feel

The Key to Safe & Effective Stretching

Here we will walk through a series of stretches that will help you understand the phrase "Go by the *feel* of the stretch." This is far more important than how *far* you stretch, or how far others stretch. This series of 6 stretches will take you 1 to 2 minutes.

Read pages 6 to 7 on how to stretch, so you understand the principles of what we are doing here.

The following stretches can be done either sitting or standing.

Note: shading indicates the areas being stretched.

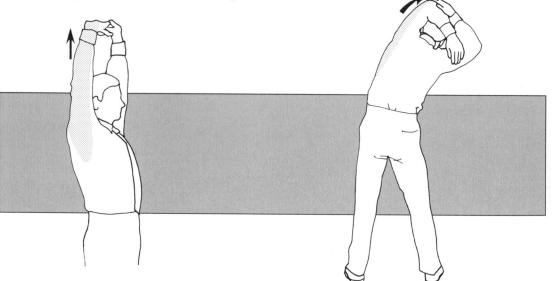

Start with knees slightly flexed. Interlace fingers over your head, reverse your hands (palms face up), and push your arms gently upward until you feel a mild stretch. Pay attention to how this feels. Don't overstretch. (You may not be able to stretch as far as shown above — don't worry about it.) Hold comfortably for 8 to 10 seconds. You should be able to say "I feel the stretch but it doesn't hurt."

Next, grasp your left elbow behind your head with your right hand until you feel a slight stretch. Then lean slightly to the right. Hold 8 to 10 seconds. Don't hold your breath; breathe easily. Then repeat for the other side: hold your right elbow with your left hand, stretch gently, and lean to the left. Don't stretch too far.

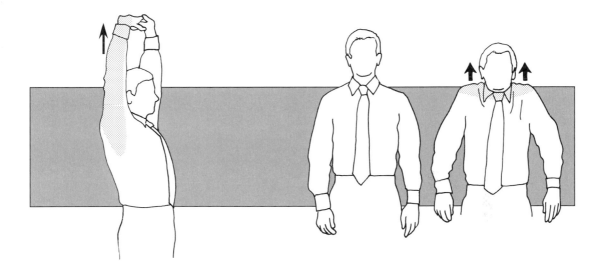

Now go back and repeat the first stretch. Knees slightly flexed, interlace fingers above head. Reverse hands and push arms gently upward. How does this *feel?* Is this stretch any easier now? Are you a little more flexible? If you do these stretches in front of a mirror, you can see how you look and also if you are stretching any farther as you go through this series.

Next raise your shoulders up toward your ear lobes with controlled tension. Hold 5–6 seconds, then relax shoulders downward. "Shoulders hang, shoulders down." Keep your jaw relaxed (your jaw should be relaxed in all the stretches).

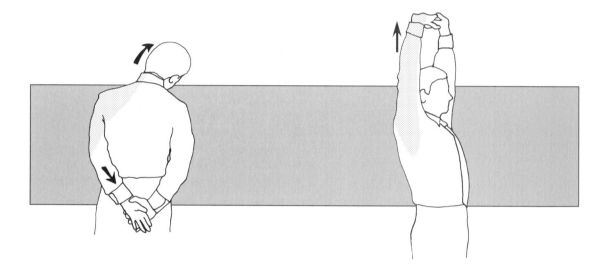

Now reach behind you and hold onto your left wrist with your right hand. Pull your right hand down and over to the right as you lean your head in the same direction. Hold 8 to 10 seconds. This stretches the neck, shoulders, and arms. Now switch and do the other side. Be sure you hold only stretches that are mild and comfortable.

Now go back and repeat the beginning stretch. With knees slightly flexed, interlace your fingers above your head. Reverse your hands and push your arms gently upward. Now how does it feel? Most people will feel more flexible in this stretch after going through this series. Again, a mirror may be helpful in showing you if you are gaining flexibility doing these stretches.

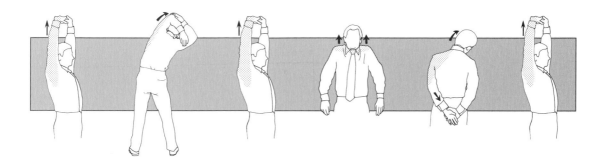

Above is a summary of the stretches we have just gone through. These are excellent to do any time at your computer to relieve neck and shoulder stiffness, to reduce stress, and to relax.

The purpose of this series of stretches has been to get you to focus on the areas being stretched, to *feel* the stretch.

Sometimes it's helpful to play with the mild tension created by the stretch. Go back and forth slowly and focus on how it feels. Go from the easy stretch into the developmental stretch *(see below)* and back again. Breathe easily, relax and concentrate on the areas being stretched.

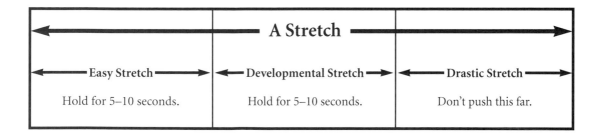

←————————————— A Stretch —————————————→		
←——— **Easy Stretch** ———→	←——— **Developmental Stretch** ———→	←——— **Drastic Stretch** ———→
Hold for 5–10 seconds.	Hold for 5–10 seconds.	Don't push this far.

Once you learn this principle, once you actually feel what stretching is doing for your muscles and tendons, you will be able to apply the principle to any stretch.

You will have learned not to overstretch. You will have learned the most important principle of stretching, which is to *go by the feel*.

Keep On Stretchin'

To stay loose, stretch regularly throughout the day. Keep this book in your desk drawer, or open on your desk (notice how the book lies flat when open).

Stretching Routines

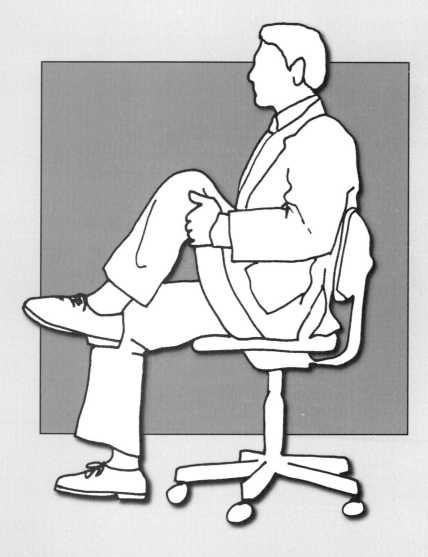

Stretching Routines

The routines that follow *(pp. 19 to 39)* are designed for easy visual reference. They are grouped by common situations, circumstances, or time of day. The important thing is to stretch regularly throughout the day.

Most of these programs take 1 to 2 minutes.

First, read the *general* stretching instructions on pages 6 to 7.

Then find the program that best suits your needs.

Lay the book open on your desk and follow the drawings. (This book's "lay-flat" binding allows it to lie flat easily.)

Each time you do a stretch for the first time, read the *specific* instructions for that stretch on pages 64 to 84. (See the page reference under each stretch.) After you follow the instructions a few times, you'll know how to do each stretch correctly. From then on, simply look at the drawings.

You may want to photocopy some of these pages to keep in your desk or on the wall.

Alternative: Another way to get started is to turn to page 65 and do the stretches one by one, following the detailed instructions. This is a good way to get familiar with each stretch.

Note: the shaded areas indicate the part of your body being stretched.

Good Morning!

Elapsed time: 1 minute

Here's a good way to start the day. While your computer is warming up, do these stretches to loosen up and get ready for work. Turn on your body while you're turning on your computer.

- Relax.
- Focus on the muscles being stretched.

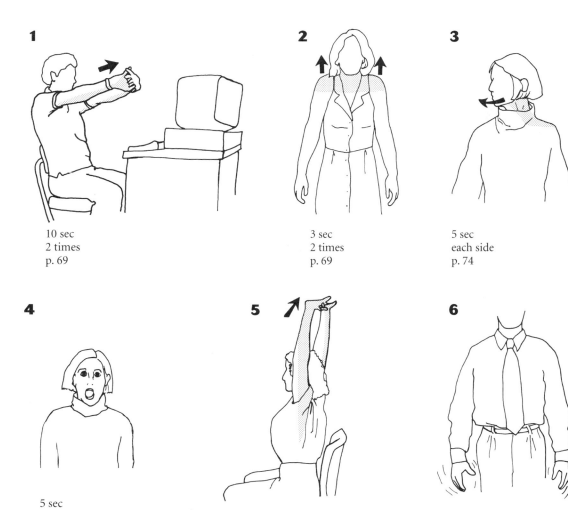

1

10 sec
2 times
p. 69

2

3 sec
2 times
p. 69

3

5 sec
each side
p. 74

4

5 sec
p. 81

5

10 sec
p. 70

6

10 sec
shake hands
p. 68

Neck & Shoulder Stiffness

Elapsed time: 1 minute

We all feel stiff from tension or holding still at the computer. Do these stretches any time of the day when you feel stiffness in the neck and/or shoulders. Each stretch takes 10 seconds or less and each one will help you relax.

- *Feel* each stretch
- Breathe easily

1

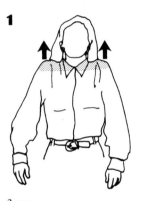

3 sec
2 times
p. 69

2

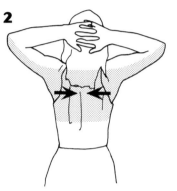

5 sec
p. 71

3

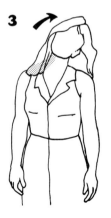

5 sec
each side
p. 73

4

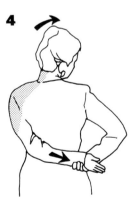

10 sec
each side
p. 72

5

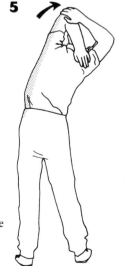

10 sec
each side
p. 70

Stretching at Your Computer or Desk © 1997 Robert A. Anderson, Jean E. Anderson & Shelter Publications, Inc.

Lower Back Stretches

Sitting for long periods is one of the biggest causes of lower back pain. Do these stretches throughout the day to move the lower back muscles and to get some circulation going. This is a good way to help avoid back problems.

Be sure to get up and move as often as possible throughout the day.

1

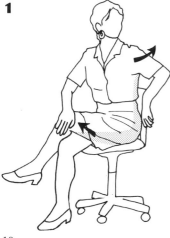

10 sec
each side
p. 80

2

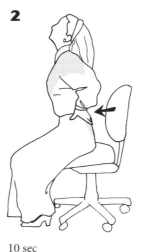

10 sec
2 times
p. 75

3

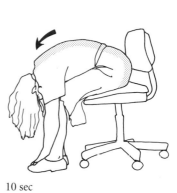

10 sec
p. 81

4

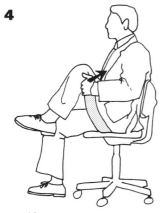

10 sec
each leg
p. 79

Caution: *If you have a history of lower back problems, consult a reliable physician who will give you tests to see exactly where the problem lies. Ask your physician which of the stretches shown in this book would be of most help to you. Also, check out the Back Revolution® on page 93; it has helped many people with back problems.*

Stretches for Keyboard Operators

Elapsed time: 76 seconds

Many people do not understand this, but working on a keyboard all day, day after day, is physically demanding. Repetitive strain injuries (RSIs) from mouse and keyboard use have risen dramatically. The routine below is specifically designed for keyboard operators and their potential (or actual) problems.

- If you are injured, see a doctor (preferably one with RSI experience) for advice on which stretches will help you recover.

- If you are not injured now, do these stretches throughout the day as preventive medicine. (Stretch while making "saves," for example.)

- *See the section, A Pain-Free Body, pp. 44 to 57, for more on RSI problems.*

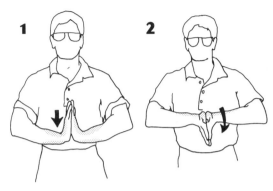

1

8 sec
p. 67

2

8 sec
p. 67

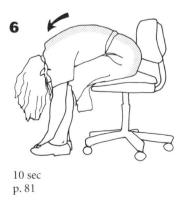

3

10 sec
2 times
p. 69

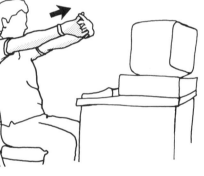

4

10–15 sec
p. 70

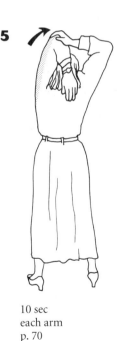

5

10 sec
each arm
p. 70

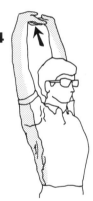

6

10 sec
p. 81

> **Move**
> *It's important to move: take a 1-minute break every 10–15 minutes, or a 5-minute break every half hour; get up and move around.*

Stretches for Graphic Artists

80 seconds

Concentrated effort on visual images puts a strain on your body as well as your eyes. Using a stylus with a drawing tablet can cause finger and wrist problems. Take frequent breaks to do these stretches, or do them while you're waiting for the computer to process information.

- Look at the stretching index on pages 94 to 95 for some other ideas.
- You can also do some exercises or move around (*see pp. 58 to 61*).

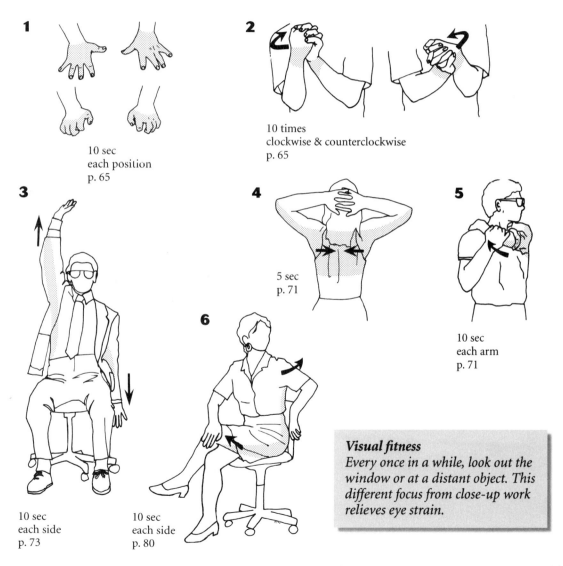

1

10 sec
each position
p. 65

2

10 times
clockwise & counterclockwise
p. 65

3

10 sec
each side
p. 73

4

5 sec
p. 71

5

10 sec
each arm
p. 71

6

10 sec
each side
p. 80

> **Visual fitness**
> *Every once in a while, look out the window or at a distant object. This different focus from close-up work relieves eye strain.*

Office Meeting Stretches

Everyone knows the physical by-products of meetings: drowsiness, stiffening, back and leg pain, etc. Try a few stretches during a meeting to counteract the effects of sitting.

See if you can educate other people in your meetings about the value of stretching. It isn't so weird!

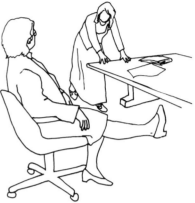

- Do these in any order.
- Breathe deeply.
- Maintain good posture.
- Every so often, tighten your abdominal muscles, pull in your stomach and hold. Then relax.
- *See index of stretches on pages 94 to 95 for other ideas.*

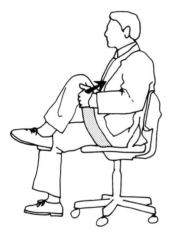

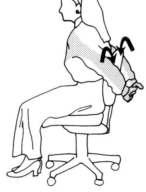

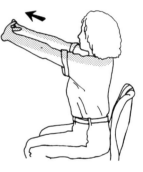

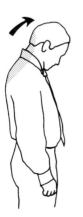

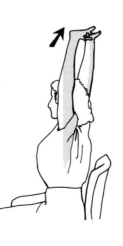

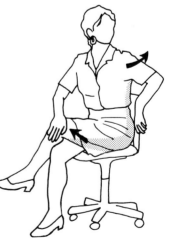

Stretching at Your Computer or Desk © 1997 Robert A. Anderson, Jean E. Anderson & Shelter Publications, Inc.

Online Stretches

1 minute

No matter how fast your modem, you're always waiting for something to load while online. (This will probably never change, for even as modems get faster and faster, files get larger and larger.) These stretches are for your upper body, especially neck, shoulders, and wrists.

- Whenever you are reading online, and not using the keyboard or mouse, you can do upper body stretches using both arms.
- After you follow this program a few times, you'll know these stretches by heart; thereafter do them frequently while online.
- Stretches 1–6 are a special routine. *See pages 10 to 13 for details.*

If there isn't time to do them all at one time, break the routine into short combinations: 1, 2, 3 or 4, 5, 6 or 7, 8.

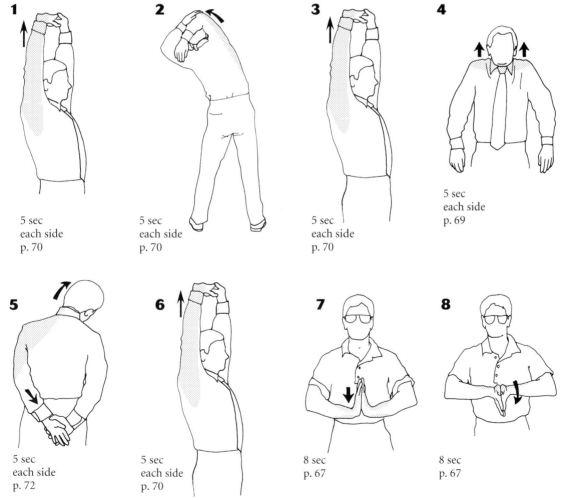

1
5 sec
each side
p. 70

2
5 sec
each side
p. 70

3
5 sec
each side
p. 70

4
5 sec
each side
p. 69

5
5 sec
each side
p. 72

6
5 sec
each side
p. 70

7
8 sec
p. 67

8
8 sec
p. 67

Stretching at Your Computer or Desk ©1997 Robert A. Anderson, Jean E. Anderson & Shelter Publications, Inc.

Stressed-Out Stretches

Elapsed time: 90 seconds

- Had a tough day?
- Computer giving you problems?
- Going to an important meeting?
- Need to relax?

There come those inevitable times during the day when the body signals it has had an overdose of stress. Don't let tension build up and ruin your good work. Pace yourself throughout the day. Take frequent stretch breaks!

- Breathe deeply.
- Take a few minutes to do these stretches.

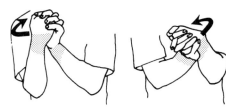

1

10 sec
each position
p. 65

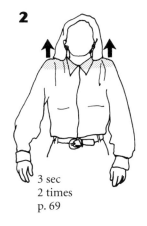
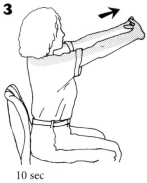

2

3 sec
2 times
p. 69

3

10 sec
2 times
p. 69

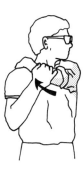

4

15 sec
each arm
p. 71

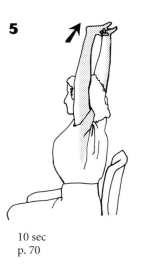

5

10 sec
p. 70

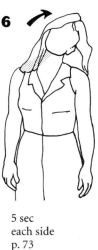

6

5 sec
each side
p. 73

Stretching at Your Computer or Desk ©1997 Robert A. Anderson, Jean E. Anderson & Shelter Publications, Inc.

Really Stressed-Out Stretches!

70 seconds

Still tense? Has it just been one of those days? In cases of advanced stress, do these stretches in addition to those on the opposite page.

- Take some more deep breaths.
- Sit quietly or meditate for a few minutes.
- Walking or any kind of movement or exercise relieves stress.
- Relax and take a few minutes for yourself!

1

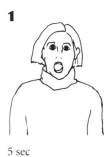

5 sec
p. 81

2

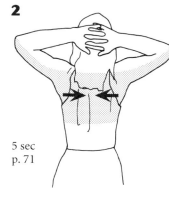

5 sec
p. 71

3

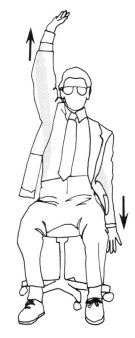

10 sec
each side
p. 73

4

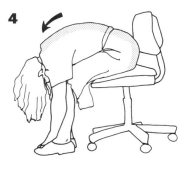

10 sec
p. 81

5

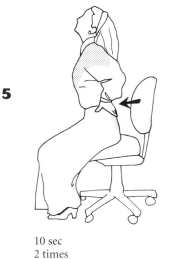

10 sec
2 times
p. 75

6

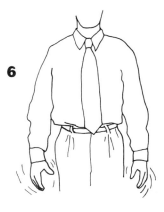

10 sec
shake hands
p. 68

Spontaneous Stretches

(Do whenever you can)

The idea here is to take a stretching break whenever you have the chance—to rejuvenate your body and recharge your energy. These stretches take only a few seconds each.

- Do these in any order.
- Pay attention to your body and stretch the parts that need it most.
- Be creative and be relaxed.
- *See stretching index on pp. 94 to 95 for other ideas.*

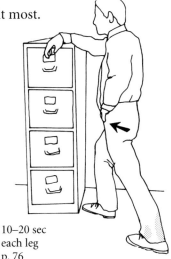

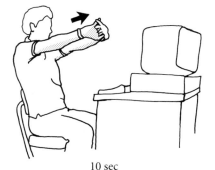

10 sec
p. 69

10–20 sec
each leg
p. 76

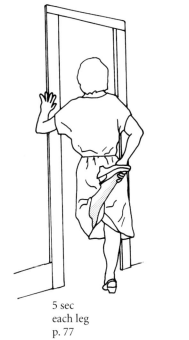

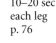

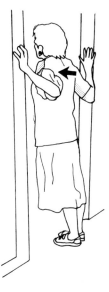

5 sec
each leg
p. 77

15 sec
each side
p. 78

15 sec
p. 75

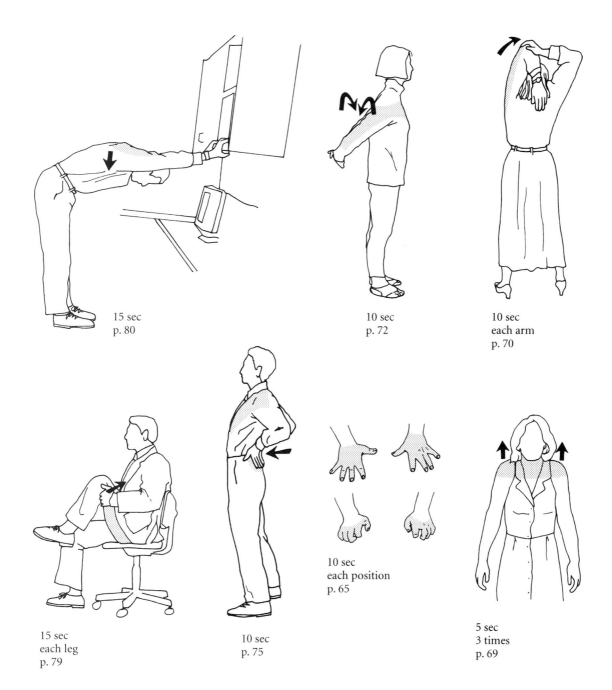

15 sec
p. 80

10 sec
p. 72

10 sec
each arm
p. 70

15 sec
each leg
p. 79

10 sec
p. 75

10 sec
each position
p. 65

5 sec
3 times
p. 69

Copy Machine Stretches

(or Waiting-for-the-Printer Stretches)

Here is a chance to stretch while you're waiting around. It's a bonus—
it doesn't take any extra time!

- Stretch while you wait for the copies.
- Do any of the stretches in this book while making copies. Be inventive!
- Copy this page on the copy machine (!) and put it on the
  wall by the copy machine.

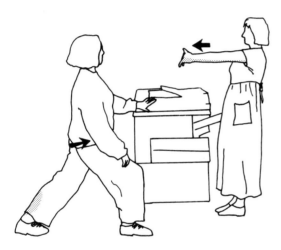

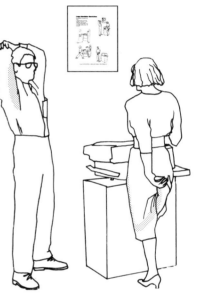

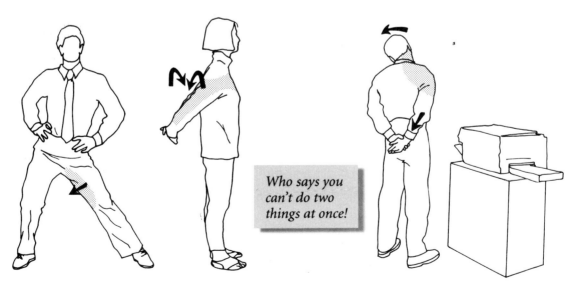

Who says you can't do two things at once!

Stretching at Your Computer or Desk ©1997 Robert A. Anderson, Jean E. Anderson & Shelter Publications, Inc.

On-the-Phone Stretches

How much time do you spend on the phone each day? All these can be done with a phone in hand. With a headset they are even easier.

- Make a copy of this page and keep it next to your phone.
- Look through the index of stretches *(pp. 94 to 95)* for ideas on other stretches to do while on the phone.

1
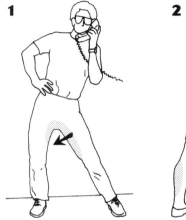

2
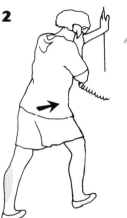

3
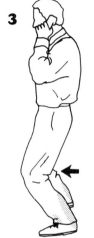

4
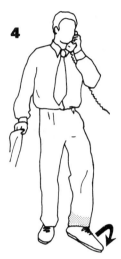

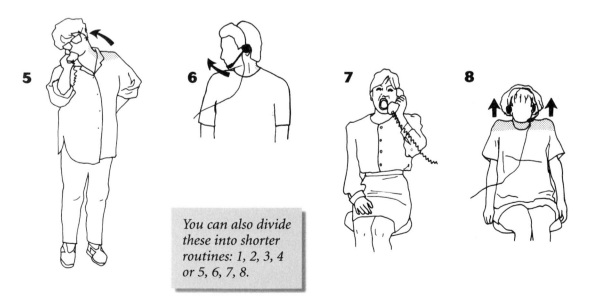

5

6

7

8

You can also divide these into shorter routines: 1, 2, 3, 4 or 5, 6, 7, 8.

Before-Walking Stretches

Elapsed time: 2 minutes

When you're ready to take a walk, even a brief one, it's wise to give your body a signal that it's about to become active; this is especially important after you have been sitting (or standing) still for a while.

Do these before taking a walk (at lunch or coffee break) or before leaving the office at night. Also, do them *after* you walk.

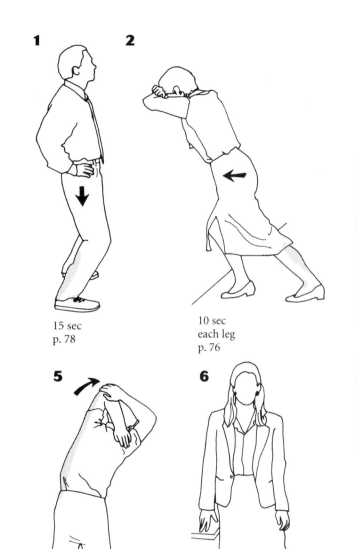

1

15 sec
p. 78

2

10 sec
each leg
p. 76

3

15 sec
each leg
p. 77

4

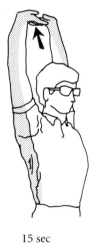

15 sec
p. 70

5

10 sec
each side
p. 70

6

8 rotations
clockwise & counterclockwise
each foot
p. 77

Adios! (Shut Down) Stretches

1 minute

Just as you take a few minutes in the morning to stretch while your computer is warming up, take 60 seconds after hitting "shut-down" before you leave the office.

- These stretches will help you shift out of the sitting mode and get you ready to move.
- Stretching is a signal to your muscles that they are about to be used.

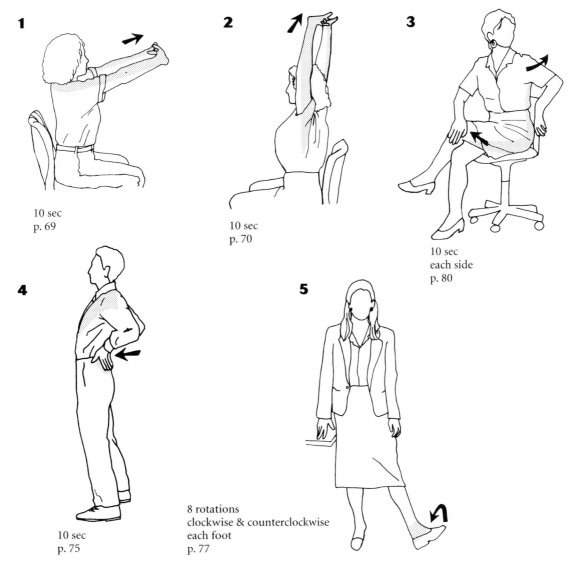

1

10 sec
p. 69

2

10 sec
p. 70

3

10 sec
each side
p. 80

4

10 sec
p. 75

5

8 rotations
clockwise & counterclockwise
each foot
p. 77

Sitting Stretches

During the hours we all spend sitting, it's beneficial to take the time to do these simple stretches. These can all be done sitting.

- Do in the order indicated.
- Do as many stretches as you like; you don't need to do them all.
- Stretch throughout the day.

1

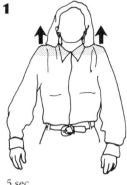

5 sec
2 times
p. 69

2

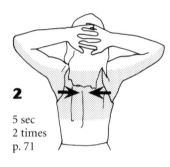

5 sec
2 times
p. 71

3

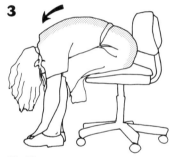

10–12 sec
p. 81

4

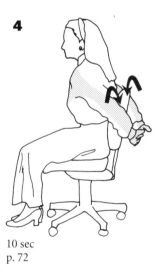

10 sec
p. 72

5

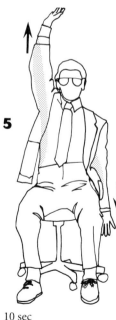

10 sec
each side
p. 73

6

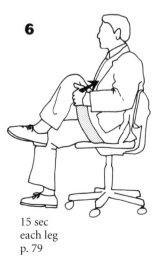

15 sec
each leg
p. 79

You can break these into shorter routines of complementary stretches: 1, 2, 3 or 4, 5, 6 or 7, 8, 9 or 10, 11, 12.

Stretching at Your Computer or Desk ©1997 Robert A. Anderson, Jean E. Anderson & Shelter Publications, Inc.

7

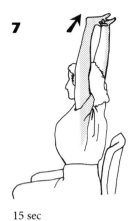

15 sec
p. 70

8

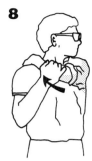

10 sec
each arm
p. 71

9

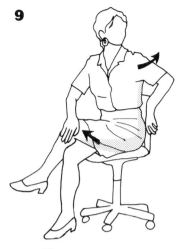

10 sec
each side
p. 80

10

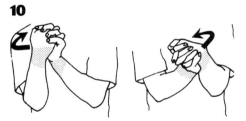

10 times
clockwise & counterclockwise
p. 65

11

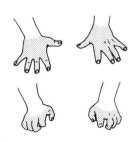

10 sec
each position
p. 65

12

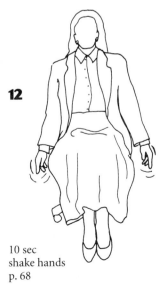

10 sec
shake hands
p. 68

Stretching at Your Computer or Desk © 1997 Robert A. Anderson, Jean E. Anderson & Shelter Publications, Inc.　　**35**

Standing Stretches

(Stand & stretch whenever possible)

Standing stretches can improve circulation (especially in your feet and legs) and relieve the neck and back stiffness that comes from prolonged sitting. It's important to get up off your behind regularly throughout the day.

- Do in the order indicated.
- Do as many stretches as you like; you don't need to do them all.
- Stretch throughout the day.

1

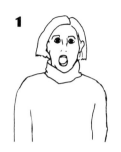

5 sec
2 times
p. 81

2

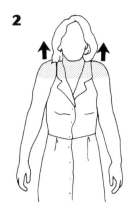

5 sec
2 times
p. 69

3

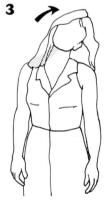

5 sec
each side
p. 73

4

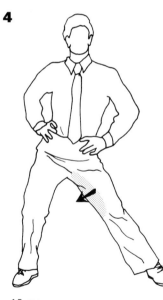

15 sec
each side
p. 78

5

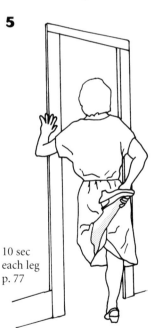

10 sec
each leg
p. 77

You can break these into shorter routines of complementary stretches: 1, 2, 3 or 4, 5, 6 or 7, 8, 9 or 10, 11, 12, 13.

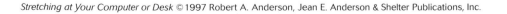

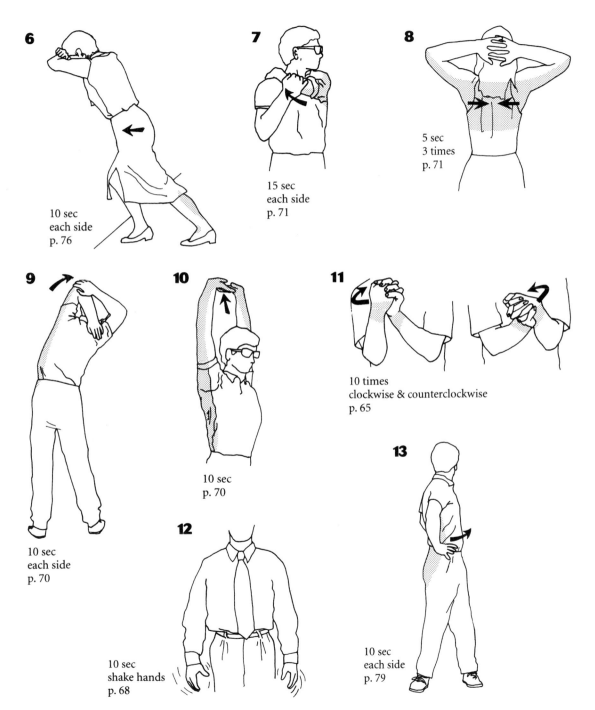

6

10 sec
each side
p. 76

7

15 sec
each side
p. 71

8

5 sec
3 times
p. 71

9

10 sec
each side
p. 70

10

10 sec
p. 70

11

10 times
clockwise & counterclockwise
p. 65

12

10 sec
shake hands
p. 68

13

10 sec
each side
p. 79

Stretching at Your Computer or Desk ©1997 Robert A. Anderson, Jean E. Anderson & Shelter Publications, Inc.

Sitting or Standing Stretches

Here is a combination of all-purpose sitting and standing stretches.

- Do in the order indicated.
- You don't have to do all these at one time; do as many stretches as you like.
- Stretch regularly throughout the day.
- Put a Post-it™ note on the bottom of your monitor as a reminder to stretch.

1

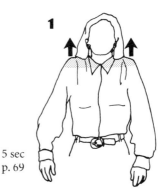

5 sec
p. 69

2

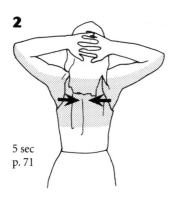

5 sec
p. 71

3

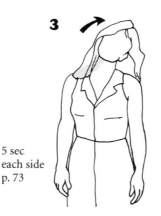

5 sec
each side
p. 73

4

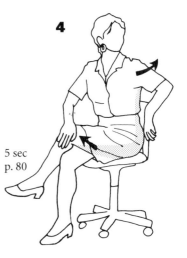

5 sec
p. 80

5

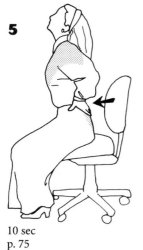

10 sec
p. 75

6

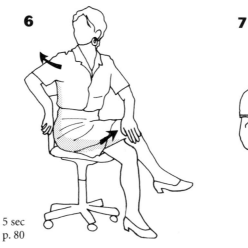

5 sec
p. 80

7

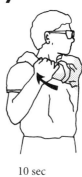

10 sec
each side
p. 71

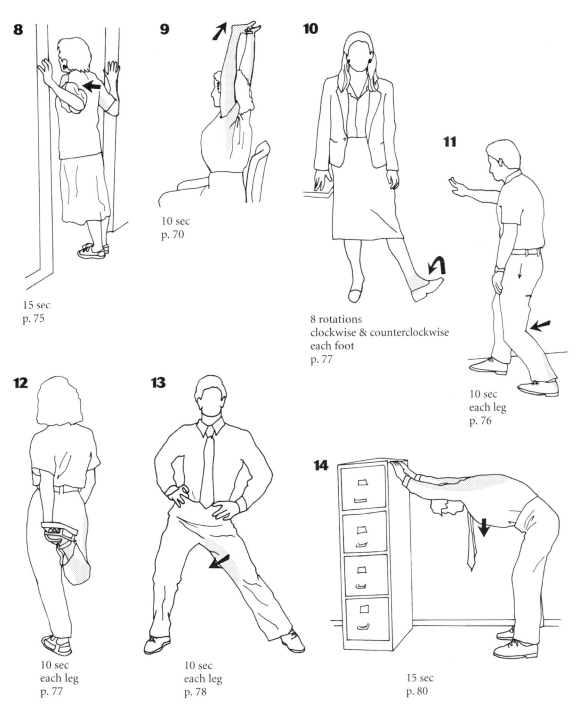

8

15 sec
p. 75

9

10 sec
p. 70

10

8 rotations
clockwise & counterclockwise
each foot
p. 77

11

10 sec
each leg
p. 76

12

10 sec
each leg
p. 77

13

10 sec
each leg
p. 78

14

15 sec
p. 80

No Gain with Pain

Hold only stretch tensions that feel good to you. Please, no forced painful stretches. They do more harm than good. The "no gain without pain" theory does not apply to stretching. Stretching *should not* be painful.

A Pain-Free Body

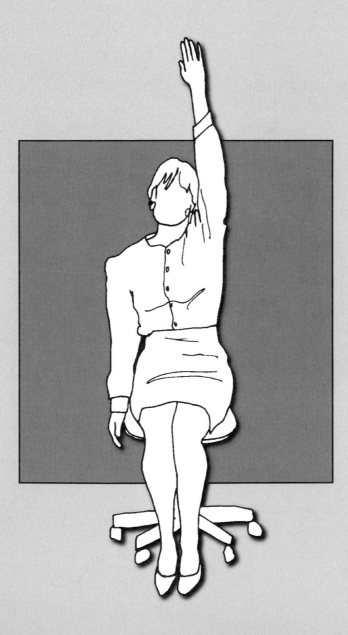

Repetitive Strain Injuries

Repetitive strain injuries (RSIs) occur from repeated physical movements that damage tendons, nerves, muscles, or other soft body tissues. Unlike sudden injuries such as broken bones or a sore back from lifting something heavy, RSIs result from a gradual, continued accumulation of small, sometimes unnoticeable, changes that eventually produce pain.

Repetitive strain, or cumulative stress injuries, are nothing new. For years, meat packers, seamstresses, assembly line workers, and others in jobs requiring continuous, repetitive physical work — especially with their hands — suffered a variety of ailments. Athletes have always had RSIs, such as runner's knee or tennis elbow.

But in the last decade a completely new category of RSI has emerged: computer-related injuries — and the problem is enormous. It is estimated that some 50 million people in the United States now use computers, and many of them work on them longer than the safe limit of three hours daily. According to the U. S. Bureau of Labor Statistics, RSIs now account for over 60% of all workplace-related illnesses, and as we head ever further into the information economy, these problems are likely to get worse.

REMEMBER TYPEWRITERS?

In the days before word processors, typists did a greater variety of manual tasks — making corrections by hand, rolling a sheet of paper in and out of the carriage, manually returning the carriage, changing ribbons. Their hands moved in a variety of directions and the brief pauses gave the wrists a rest. With computers, however, these activities are automated. The operator may perform over 20,000 keystrokes in a single work period, with no variation and no "wrist rest" time.

ELECTRONIC INJURIES

Recent increases in computer usage and flat, light-touch keyboards that permit high-speed typing have resulted in an epidemic of injuries to the hands, arms, and shoulders. Pointing devices such as a mouse or a trackball are in large part responsible. Slowly, the thousands of repeated keystrokes and long periods of clutching and dragging with a mouse damage the body. Another name for these problems is Cumulative Trauma Disorder. This happens even more quickly due to improper keyboarding technique and/or body positions that place unnecessary stress on the tendons and nerves in the hand, wrist, arms, and even the shoulders and neck. Lack of adequate rest, not taking breaks, or using excessive force almost guarantee trouble.

CARPAL TUNNEL SYNDROME, ET AL

You may have heard the term *Carpal Tunnel Syndrome* (CTS) in connection with these injuries, but in fact CTS represents only a small and dangerous percentage of typing injuries. In his book *Repetitive Strain Injury,* Emil Pascarelli, M.D., states that DeQuervain's disease, involving acute pain at the junction of wrist and thumb, is a more common (if less known) problem than CTS. There are various types of tendinitis (shoulder, forearm, etc.), different forms of nerve damage, shoulder problems from holding the phone with one raised shoulder while typing, elbow and wrist problems from using the mouse, loss of circulation in the fingers, and different types of arthritis that may be aggravated by cumulative stress. All of these are serious and, in advanced cases, can cause great pain and permanent disability. It is not uncommon for people to have to leave computer-dependent careers as a result.

THINGS TO WATCH FOR

- Tightness, discomfort, stiffness, or pain in the hands, wrists, fingers, forearms, or elbows

- Tingling, coldness, or numbness in the hands

- Clumsiness or loss of strength and coordination in the hands

- Recurring pain in the neck or shoulders

- Pain that wakes you up at night

WHAT IF YOU HAVE SUCH SYMPTOMS?

We all have occasional aches and pains that go away in a day or two. But if you have recurring problems from using the computer, run, do not walk, to your doctor or health care provider *right away*. An early diagnosis is critical to limiting the damage, and may spare you a world of hurt, trouble, and frustration. You are not overreacting: by the time you have symptoms, some damage has already been done. If you try to ignore the pain, you may sustain a serious injury. If your doctor doesn't seem to know much about RSIs, find one who does. When you find one, listen to the diagnosis and get advice on any changes you intend to make or therapy you intend to try. There are no quick fixes. No wrist splint, arm rest, split keyboard, spinal adjustment, etc. is going to get you right back to work at full speed if you've been injured. Even carpal tunnel sufferers who undergo the release surgery on their wrists can be back in pain and trouble if they don't make long-term changes in the technique and work habits that hurt them in the first place. Healing *does* happen but it takes months, not days.

Ergonomic Principles

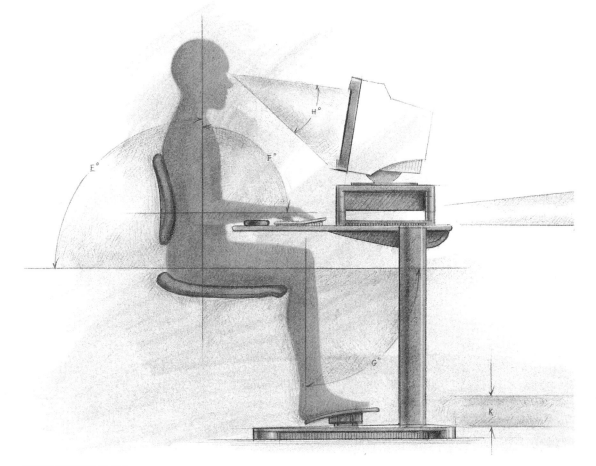

ERGONOMICS

The term *ergonomics* comes from the Greek words *ergos* meaning "work" and *nomos,* meaning "study of" or "natural laws of." The science of ergonomics dates back to the 1940s, but only in the past decade has it become a commonly known term. This is due to the recent epidemic of office-related injuries and the large body of equipment and information designed to solve these problems.

Modern-day office ergonomics is the science of providing furniture, tools, and equipment that improve the comfort, safety, and health of the office worker. We are not ergonomic experts, but we have studied the literature on the subject and there seem to be some basic principles on which most professionals agree. The following 4 pages contain some of the basics as an introduction to the subject.

SOME ERGONOMIC SPECIFICS

- **Monitor** should be an arm's length or a bit more from your eyes. Conventional ergonomic wisdom generally advises people that the center of the screen should be where their gaze falls naturally, with the top of the screen at eye level, and that the monitor should be tilted slightly to match the angle of one's gaze. A 1995 report, *Vision Comfort at VDTs,* by Stewart B. Leavitt, however, comes to a different conclusion: the monitor should be lower than this, in a *range* with the top about 15° below horizontal eye level to the lower limit where the bottom of the screen is 45° below eye level. If you are concerned about vision comfort and especially if you have eye problems such as blurring vision, burning eyes, or even neck and shoulder pain, we recommend that you read this detailed report *(see p. 88)*. An adjustable stand or monitor riser (or homemade box) will allow you to make adjustments.

- **Keyboard** should be set at a height so that forearms, wrists, and hands are aligned when keyboarding, and parallel to the floor, or bent slightly down from elbow to hand—the hands are never bent back. Preferably the stand or desk on which the keyboard sits is adjustable. There are many "ergonomic" keyboards available, some of them quite unusual.

- **Mouse pad** should be at a height where your arm, wrist, and hand are aligned and in "neutral." It is best if the stand or desk the mouse pad sits on is adjustable.

- **Wrists,** while you are actually typing, should not rest on anything, and should not be bent up, down, or to the side. Your arms should move your hands around, and instead of resting your wrists, you should stretch to hit keys with your fingers. (There are wrist-rest devices on the market that give you a place to rest your hands, but only when pausing from typing, not *while* you are typing.)

- **Chair** should be adjustable and comfortable. Set it so that your thighs are either parallel to the floor or at a slight downward angle from the hips to the knees. You should sit straight, not slouching, and not straining forward to reach the keys. Stay relaxed. Anything that creates awkward reaches or angles in the body will create problems.

FURTHER TIPS

- **Align your wrists** Wrists also should not be bent to the side; instead your fingers should be in a straight line with your forearm, as viewed from above.

- **The proper keyboard angle** Research suggests that it may be better to tilt the back edge of your keyboard down, away from you. Put a prop an inch or two thick under the edge of the keyboard closest to you, but make sure the whole thing is still low enough so you aren't reaching up.

• **Frequently change positions** Movement is important during the working day. You may want to adjust the height or angle of your chair after a few hours, or to stand after sitting for a period. In fact, as reported in the ergonomic newsletter *OccuTrax* (Black Mountain, NC), "Ergonomic studies have verified that the least stressful working position is one where the individual can 'sit and stand' rather than sit 'or' stand."

• **Don't pound the keys** Use a light touch.

• **Use two hands to perform double-key operations** such as Command-P, Ctrl-C or Alt-F, instead of twisting one hand to do them. Move your whole hand to hit function keys with your strong fingers instead of stretching to reach them.

• **Hold the mouse lightly** Don't grip it hard or squeeze it. Place it where you don't have to reach up or over very far to use it (close to the keyboard is best). Better yet: learn and use equivalent keyboard commands whenever possible, as no pointing device is risk-free. Even trackballs have injured users.

• **Keep your arms and hands warm** Cold muscles and tendons are at much greater risk for overuse injuries, and many offices are overly air-conditioned.

• **Rest** When you stop typing for a while, rest your hands in your lap and/or on their sides instead of leaving them on the keyboard.

• **Stretch** Stretch frequently throughout the day *(see pages 52 to 55)*.

• **Move** Get up and move whenever you can. If possible, walk to talk to a near-by colleague instead of using the phone. Try using the stairs (at least for some floors) instead of the elevator.

• **Take breaks** Holding utterly still is deadly. Some experts suggest a 10-second break every 3 minutes, others suggest a 1-minute break every 15 minutes, a 5-minute break every half hour, or a 15-minute break every 2 hours, etc. You can stretch and/or move around during these breaks.

• **Eliminate unnecessary computer usage.** No ergonomic changes, fancy keyboards, or exercises are going to help if you are typing more than your body can handle. Ask yourself: can some electronic-mail messages be replaced by telephone calls? How much time are you spending on the Internet? And watch it on the computer video games, which often involve long, unbroken sessions of very tense keyboard or controller use. If nothing else, *pause* the game every 3 to 4 minutes. Don't sacrifice your hands to a game!

TAKE CARE OF YOUR EYES

Anyone who operates a computer regularly would be wise to get a complete eye exam. Even minor sight defects should be corrected with lenses designed specifically for computer usage. Many computer operators, if they do not have to focus on distant objects while keyboarding, utilize bifocal lenses with the top calibrated for the computer screen and the bottom for reading. Or, if distant vision is required, the bifocals can have the top designed for distance and the bottom for the computer. Progressive lenses are also an option, where magnification is a gradient from top to bottom.

Glare on the screen should be avoided. A glare hood may help if there are overhead lights.Try to have any windows to the side, not in front of or behind the computer.

It's also very important to look up from the screen periodically and to focus on a distant object for a minute or two; do some stretches while doing this.

For further information see the description of Vision Comfort at VDTs— The Ergonomic Positioning of Monitors and Word Documents *on page 88.*

VOICE-RECOGNITION TECHNOLOGY

Voice recognitions systems allow you to input information with your voice or in conjunction with the keyboard and mouse. These entail software, and in some cases, hardware, and are very important for people who can no longer use a keyboard. (They can also be extremely useful while healing takes place.) *See references to the* Onsight Ergonomic Products Resources Guide *on page 91 and also the* Typing Injury FAQ Website *on page 91 in the Bibliography.*

THE ENVIRONMENT

Lighting, wall color, ventilation, reflections, electromagnetic fields, sounds, air quality, view, and other factors are all important considerations in an office environment. There are many sources of information on this topic you can investigate. *(See pp. 88 to 91 for resources.)*

WHAT CAN STRETCHING DO?

The author is not a doctor nor a specialist in injuries of any kind. However, from teaching people to stretch for over 20 years, he has seen the value of stretching in just about every area of physical activity. Here is what he would suggest:

- *If you are not injured,* use the stretches on pages 52 to 55 as preventative medicine. These are shoulder, neck, arm, hand, and wrist stretches. Stretch regularly throughout the day and you may be able to avoid RSI.

- *If you are injured,* take this book to your doctor or health care provider and ask which of the stretching programs you can follow. Point out that the stretching index on pages 94 to 95 can be used to customize a series of stretches for your particular condition.

THE VALUE OF EXERCISE

Exercise can help in just about every type of physical problem. For ideas on how to work some movement into your daily office schedule, see page 60.

FURTHER REFERENCE

On pages 88 to 91, we list books on RSI, ergonomics, catalogs with extensive product lines, and addresses for the large amount of information available on the Internet. You can also check the ads in your Yellow Pages under Office Furniture; look for the word "ergonomic."

Healing Takes Time

If you have a repetitive strain injury, don't expect an instant cure. Many people have found that after a few months of following good ergonomic principles *(see pp. 46 to 50)* and stretching regularly, their condition has improved.

Hand, Arm, Shoulder & Neck Stretches

(To Prevent Repetitive Strain Injuries)

Here is a series of stretches for the hands, arms, shoulders, and neck. If you have RSI-type problems, do not do any of these that cause pain. *Proceed with caution.*

If you do not have an RSI-type problem, we recommend you follow this routine as *preventive medicine.*

1

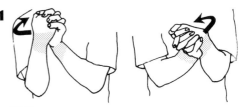

10 times
clockwise & counterclockwise
p. 65

2

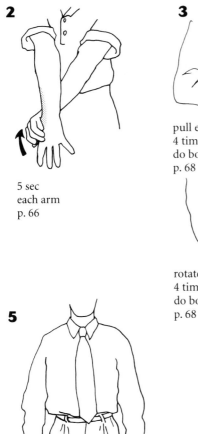

5 sec
each arm
p. 66

3

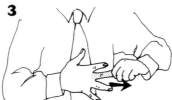

pull each finger & thumb gently
4 times each direction
do both hands
p. 68

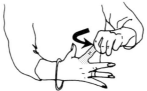

rotate each finger & thumb gently
4 times each direction
do both hands
p. 68

4

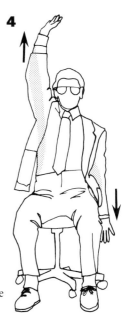

10 sec
each side
p. 73

5

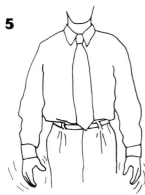

10 sec
shake hands
p. 68

6

5 sec
3 times
p. 69

Stretching at Your Computer or Desk © 1997 Robert A. Anderson, Jean E. Anderson & Shelter Publications, Inc.

- *Alternative.* You can do all 13 stretches in the order indicated; this will take 2 to 3 minutes. Or if you don't have time to do all of these at one time, you can break them into shorter routines of complementary stretches: 1, 2, 3 or 4, 5, 6, 7 or 8, 9,10 or 11, 12, 13.
- Frequently, the cause of wrist and hand problems is in the neck, shoulders or arms.
- The most important thing is to stretch regularly throughout the day.
- "An ounce of prevention . . ."

7

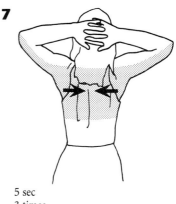
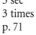

5 sec
3 times
p. 71

8

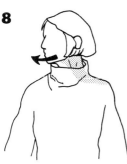

5 sec
2 times
each side
p. 74

9

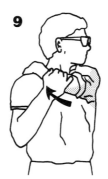

10 sec
each side
p. 71

10

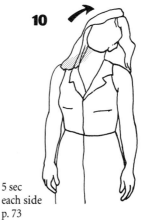

5 sec
each side
p. 73

11

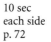

10 sec
2 times
p. 69

12

10 sec
p. 70

13

10 sec
each side
p. 72

Hand, Wrist & Forearm Stretches

(To Prevent Repetitive Strain Injuries)

Here is a series of stretches for the hands, wrists and forearms. If you have RSI-type problems, do not do any of these that cause pain. *Proceed with caution.*

If you do not have an RSI-type problem, we recommend you follow this routine as *preventive medicine.*

1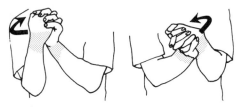

10 times
clockwise & counterclockwise
p. 65

2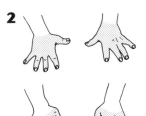

10 sec
each position
p. 65

3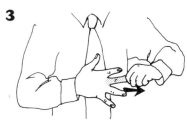

pull each finger & thumb gently
4 times each direction, do both hands
p. 68

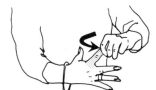

rotate each finger & thumb gently
4 times each direction, do both hands
p. 68

4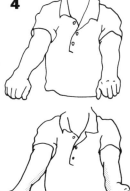

5 sec
2 times
p. 66

5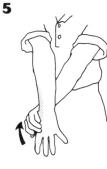

5 sec
each arm
p. 66

6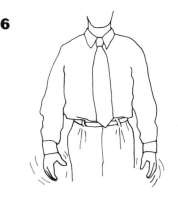

10 sec
shake hands
p. 68

7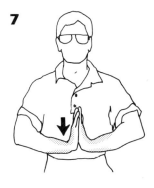

10 sec
p. 67

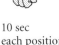

Wrist Stretches

Here is a special series of stretches for the wrists. You can do one or more of these at any time, especially while waiting a few seconds for the computer to process information. If you have wrist problems, do not do any of these that cause pain. If you do not have wrist problems, use these as *preventive medicine.*

- These are especially helpful stretches if you do a lot of keyboarding.
- Keep your wrists flexible and fingers supple.

1

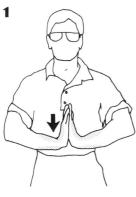

8 sec
p. 67

2

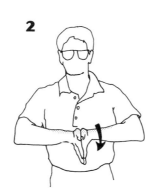

8 sec
p. 67

3

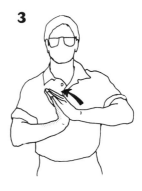

5 sec
each wrist
p. 67

4

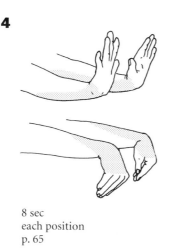

8 sec
each position
p. 65

5

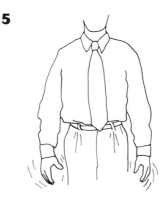

10 sec
shake hands
p. 68

Good Habits for a Pain-Free Body

Posture and body position are extremely important in anything you do. Here are some brief tips on sitting, standing, and lifting. Open the book to these pages every so often and practice these suggestions until you eventually train your body to do them automatically.

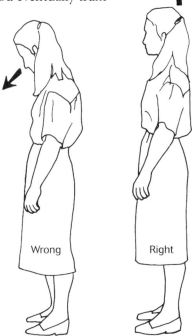

Wrong   Right

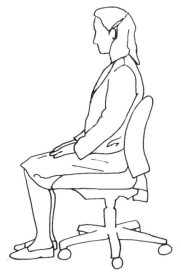

Sitting Posture

An "ergonomic" chair with a firm back and support enables you to maintain the lumbar curve in your low back. Set the chair at a proper level so that your knees are level when both feet are flat on floor. Don't cross your legs. Don't lean forward or slouch. Note: crossing your ankles is better for circulation than crossing your knees. (See page 46 for more information on sitting.)

Standing Posture

- When standing, bend knees slightly; don't lock knees—keeping them slightly bent gives you some spring, some flex.
- Use your quadriceps muscles to control your posture when standing. This is a position of power.
- Keeping your pelvis slightly pushed forward and your stomach tucked in will help prevent lower back pain.
- Imagine a string coming out of the top of your head and from which you hang; this helps you visualize proper alignment.

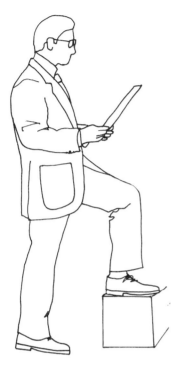

Standing

When you stand in one place for a period of time, prop one foot up on a box or a short stool. Alternate your feet often. This will relieve some of the back tension that comes from prolonged standing.

Lifting

- Hold the lifted load close to your body. The closer you hold it, the less stress on your back.
- Keep your back upright during the lift.
- Bend your knees and minimize any bending at the waist. Bending at the waist, with legs straight, greatly increases the strain on your back.
- Lift with your legs by slowly straightening them. Make your legs do the work, not your back.
- Don't twist while lifting.

Office Exercises

By Bill Pearl

Sirtting much of the day causes loss of muscle tone due to inactivity. Here are a few light muscle-strengthening exercises from four-time Mr. Universe Bill Pearl. They can be done in the office with no equipment. (This is weight training without the weights—using only your body weight.) Use your imagination for other things you can do.

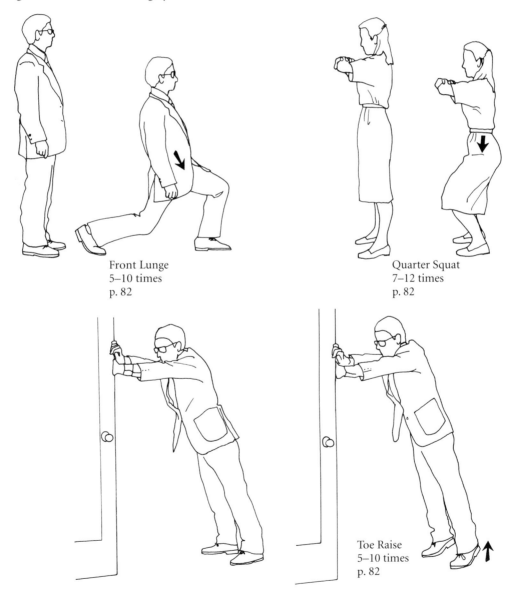

Front Lunge
5–10 times
p. 82

Quarter Squat
7–12 times
p. 82

Toe Raise
5–10 times
p. 82

Stretching at Your Computer or Desk © 1997 Robert A. Anderson, Jean E. Anderson & Shelter Publications, Inc.

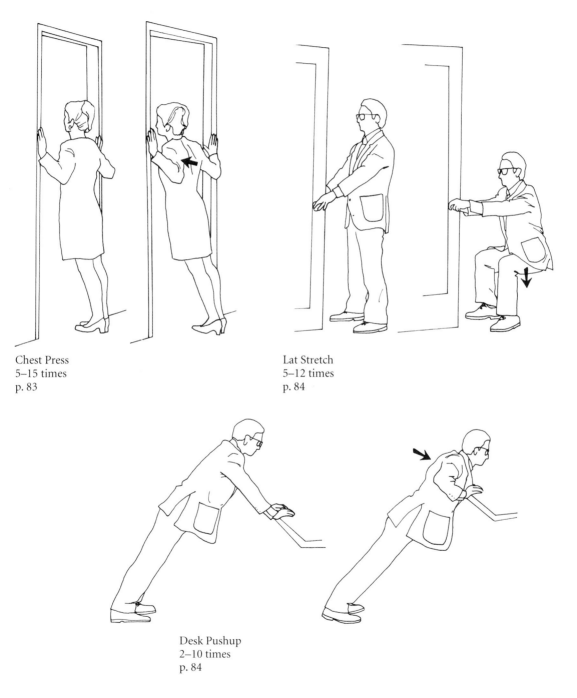

Chest Press
5–15 times
p. 83

Lat Stretch
5–12 times
p. 84

Desk Pushup
2–10 times
p. 84

Moving

THE ANTIDOTE FOR SITTING

Sitting for long periods is a very recent phenomenon in human history. Many health problems of the modern world are either caused by or aggravated by the sedentary life.

In recent years, exercise has been shown to have beneficial effects for a variety of medical problems. From arthritis to back pain (the recommendation used to be "stay in bed") to osteoporosis to cancer. Likewise, moving exercise can help decrease the chances of contracting office-related injuries and, if done sensibly, can help heal symptoms and speed recovery.

THE NEW APPROACH

In the last two decades, there has been an overemphasis on strenuous workouts in America. Running marathons, intense aerobic dance classes, competitive cycling, and swimming were often touted as necessary for good health. Experience has shown, however, that most people will not stick with an exercise program that is too strenuous. More recent studies show that even mild exercise, such as walking 10 minutes a day, can do a world of good. Or as Dr. Steven Blair puts it in his book *Living With Exercise,* "Standing is better than sitting, moving is better than standing . . ." If you have been sedentary for some time, try walking 5 minutes; then the next day 6 minutes, and so on. Or walk around the house during TV commercials.

Here are a few ideas for building some physical activity into your daily life.

ON THE JOB

- *Take mini-walks* Walk during coffee breaks. Arrange a walk-and-talk instead of a sit-and-talk meeting.

- *Climb stairs* Walk at least some of the distance up or down in office buildings.

- *Park and walk* Park farther away from the office (or the store when shopping), instead of trying to get as close as possible.

- *Walk on your lunch break* You'll return refreshed. Wear comfortable shoes.

- *Move while on the phone* Stand and move around while talking on the phone. Do some stretches. *(See p. 31.)*

- Swing your arms, turn your neck, or wiggle your toes — any kind of movement helps.

OFF THE JOB

Use off-the-job time to exercise neglected muscles rather than straining those that are already overworked. Be creative.

- *Walking* is now the most popular form of exercise in America. It can be done practically anytime, anywhere and all you need is a good pair of shoes.

- *Walk with the kid(s)* when babysitting.

- *Games* are a great way to exercise. Softball, volleyball, bowling, tennis, any of these things you do for fun and socializing will get your circulation going.

- *Dancing* is also great exercise and fun.

- *House and garden work* such as mowing the lawn, vacuuming the house, washing the car, etc. are all moving exercise.

- *Regular exercise* Any typical endurance activity such as running, cycling, swimming, especially if done 3 times a week, will do you a world of good.

Stretch and Move at Work So You Have a Life When You Get Home

Many people feel awful after work and don't feel like doing anything then. However, if you can stretch, and do a little walking or other exercise in the office, you'll feel better when you get home. You'll have more energy to do things that are fun and/or fitness-oriented.

Stretching Instructions

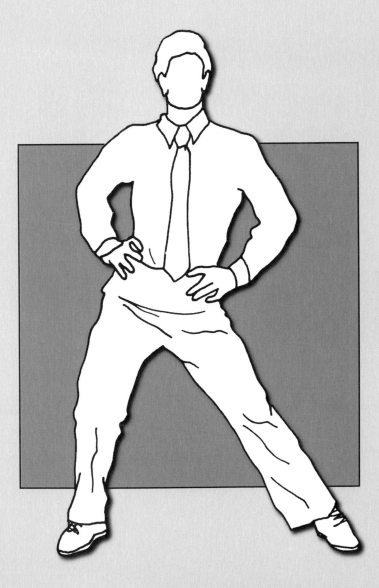

Detailed Instructions on How to Do Each Stretch

In this section there are 43 different stretches and exercises with detailed instructions telling you how to do each one. It's important to know the proper procedures and positions for the stretches, even though they are simple. You'll get the full benefits of stretching by doing the stretches correctly.

- Each stretch in the routines *(pp. 19 to 55)* has a page number reference to these instructions.

- Refer to the instructions until you know what to do for each stretch. From then on, you'll only have to look at the figures in the programs.

- *An alternative to the routines:* You can also follow through these instructions, one after the other, rather than using the routines on pages 19 to 55.

- ***Note:*** *The shading in each drawing shows those areas of the body where you will most likely feel the stretch.*

Hands & Wrists

- Separate and straighten your fingers until the tension of a stretch is felt
- Hold 10 seconds
- Relax, then bend fingers at the knuckles and hold 10 seconds
- Repeat the first stretch once more

Stretches hands, fingers, and wrists

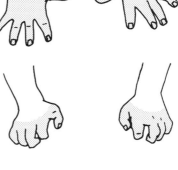

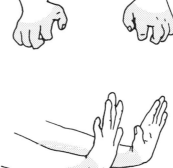

- With arms extended, palms down, bend your wrists and raise your fingertips
- Hold 10 seconds
- Now bend your wrists back in the opposite direction, fingers pointing down
- Hold 10 seconds

Stretches wrists and lower arms

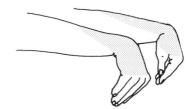

- Interlace your fingers in front of you
- Rotate your hands and wrists clockwise 10 times
- Repeat counterclockwise 10 times

Stretches wrists

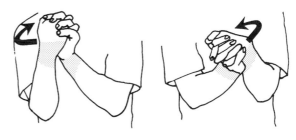

- With right arm held straight out, turn palm of hand up
- Reach under forearm with your left hand and hold your thumb and inside of palm
- With your left hand, slowly turn your right hand out and down until you feel a mild stretch
- Hold 5–10 seconds
- Repeat for other arm

Stretches wrists and forearms

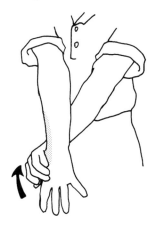

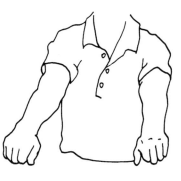

- Arms straight out in front
- Slowly turn your hands to the outside until a stretch is felt
- Hold 5–10 seconds

Stretches wrists and forearms

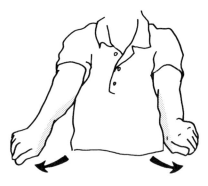

- Place your hands palm-to-palm in front of you
- Move hands downward, keeping your palms together, until you feel a mild stretch
- Keep elbows up and even
- Hold 5–8 seconds

Stretches wrists, forearms, and hands

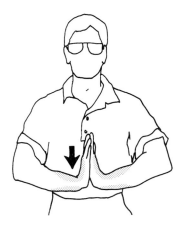

- From above stretch, rotate palms around until they face more or less downward
- Go until you feel a mild stretch
- Keep elbows up and even
- Hold 5–8 seconds

Stretches wrists, forearms, and hands

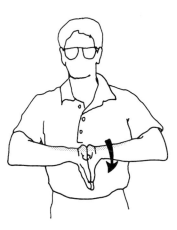

- Place your hands palm-to-palm in front of you
- Push one hand gently to the side until you feel a mild stretch
- Keep elbows up and even
- Hold 5–8 seconds

Stretches wrists, forearms, and hands

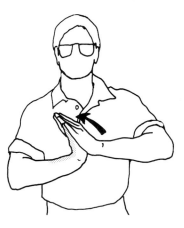

Hands

- Hold the index finger of your opposite hand
- Rotate 5 times clockwise, then 5 times counterclockwise
- Rotate each finger and thumb

Stretches fingers

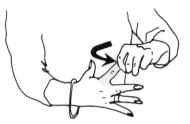

- Next, gently pull your finger straight out and hold 2–3 seconds
- Do the same thing with each finger and thumb
- Repeat for your other hand

Stretches fingers

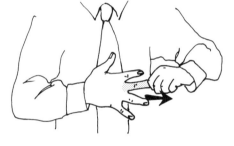

- Shake your arms and hands at your sides 10–12 seconds
- Keep your jaw relaxed and let shoulders hang downward as you shake out the tension

Increases circulation

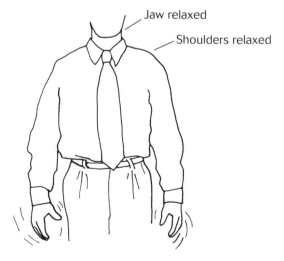

Jaw relaxed

Shoulders relaxed

Shoulders & Arms

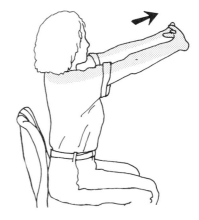

- Interlace your fingers, then straighten your arms out in front of you
- Palms should be facing away from you
- Feel the stretch in your arms and through the upper part of your back (shoulder blades)
- Hold stretch 10 seconds

Stretches shoulders, arms, wrists, and fingers

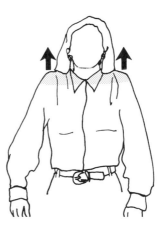

This is a good stretch to use at the first signs of tightness or tension in the shoulder and neck area.

- Raise the top of your shoulders toward your ears until you feel a slight tension in your neck and shoulders
- Hold this 3–5 seconds, then relax your shoulders downward into normal position
- Think: "shoulders hang, shoulders down"

Stretches shoulders and neck

- Hold your left elbow with your right hand
- Gently pull your elbow behind your head until an easy tension-stretch is felt in shoulder or back of your upper arm (triceps)
- Hold easy stretch 10 seconds
- Don't overstretch or hold breath
- Do both sides

Stretches triceps, top of shoulders, and sides

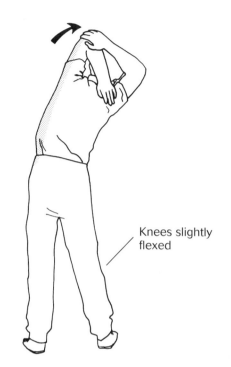

Knees slightly flexed

- Interlace your fingers, then turn your palms upward above your head as you straighten your arms
- Think of elongating your arms as you feel a stretch through your arms and upper sides of your rib cage
- Hold 10–15 seconds
- Excellent for slumping shoulders
- Breathe deeply

Stretches shoulders, back, arms, and hands

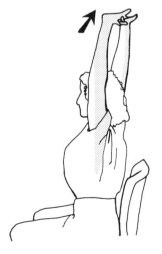

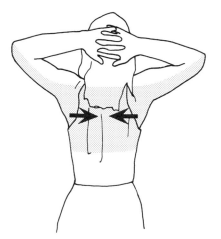

- With fingers interlaced behind your head, keep your elbows straight out to the side with your upper body erect
- Now pull your shoulder blades toward each other to create a feeling of tension through your upper back and shoulder blades
- Hold 5 seconds, then relax

Stretches shoulders, chest, and upper back

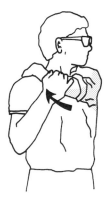

- Hold your left arm just above your elbow with your right hand
- As you look over your left shoulder, gently pull your elbow toward the opposite shoulder until a stretch is felt
- Hold 10–15 seconds
- Do both sides

Stretches sides of shoulders, back of upper arms, and neck

Shoulders & Arms

- Interlace your fingers behind your back, palms facing your back
- Slowly turn your elbows inward while straightening your arms until a stretch is felt
- Lift your breast bone slightly upward as you stretch
- Hold 10 seconds

Stretches arms, chest, hands, and shoulders

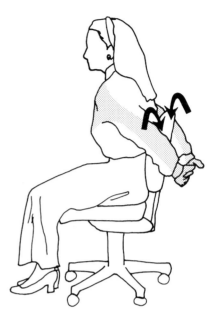

- With your right hand, gently pull your left arm gently down and across, behind your back
- Lean your head sideways toward the right shoulder
- Hold 10 seconds
- Repeat other side
- Relax

Stretches top of shoulders and neck

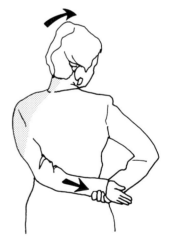

Shoulders, Arms & Neck

- Extend your right arm above your head

- Reach down with your left arm as you reach up with your right arm

- Point your fingers

- Hold 10 seconds

- Repeat other side

- If you do this stretch standing, keep your knees slightly flexed

- Breathe easily

Stretches shoulders and arms

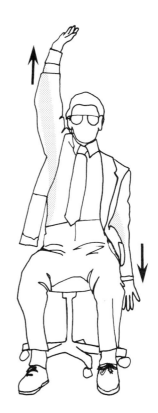

- Sit or stand, arms hanging loosely at your sides

- Tilt your head sideways, first to one side, then the other

- Keep your shoulders relaxed downward during the stretch

- Hold 5 seconds each side

Stretches sides of neck

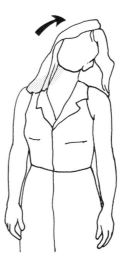

Neck & Shoulders

- Sit or stand with your arms hanging loosely at your sides
- Gently tilt your head forward to stretch the back of your neck
- Keep your shoulders relaxed downward
- Hold 5 seconds

Stretches neck

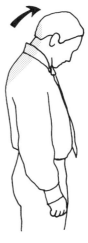

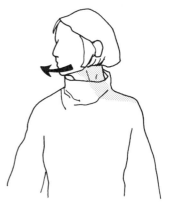

- Sit or stand with your arms hanging loosely at your sides
- Turn your head to one side, then to the other
- Hold 5 seconds, each side

Stretches sides of neck

- Place hands just above the back of your hips, elbows back
- Gently press forward
- Slightly lift your breast bone upward as you hold the stretch
- Hold 10–15 seconds
- Breathe easily
- *Note: can also be done sitting*

Stretches chest and back

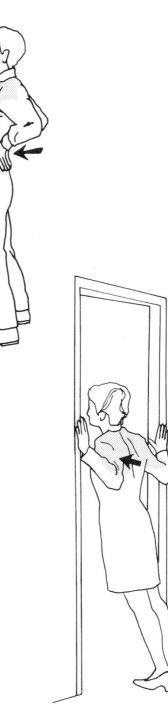

- Place your hands at shoulder-height on either side of a doorway
- Move your upper body forward until you feel a comfortable stretch
- Keep your chest and head up, your knees slightly bent
- Hold 15 seconds
- Breathe easily

Stretches chest and inside of upper arms

Legs

- Stand a little way from a wall and lean on it with your forearms, head resting on your hands
- Place your right foot in front of you, your leg bent, your left leg straight behind you
- Slowly move your hips forward until you feel a stretch in the calf of your left leg
- Keep your left heel flat and toes pointed straight ahead
- Hold easy stretch 10–20 seconds
- Do not bounce
- Repeat other leg

Stretches calves

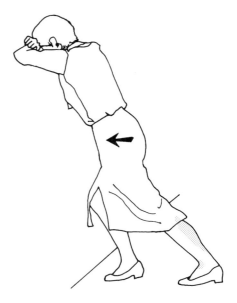

- From the previous stretch, lower your hips downward
- Slightly bend your left knee, keeping your back flat
- Keep your left foot slightly toed-in or straight, heel down
- Hold 10 seconds
- Repeat other leg

Stretches calves, Achilles area, and ankles

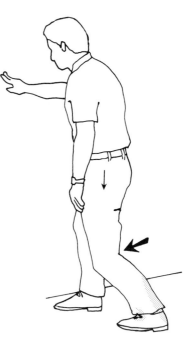

- Stand and hold onto something for balance
- Lift your left foot and rotate foot and ankle 8–10 times clockwise, then 8–10 times counterclockwise
- Repeat other side
- *Note: can also be done sitting*

Stretches ankles and improves circulation

- Place your right hand on something for support (e.g., wall or chair)
- Standing straight, grasp the top of your right foot with your left hand
- Gently pull your heel toward your buttock until a slight stretch is felt
- Hold 10–20 seconds
- Repeat for other leg

Stretches front of thighs (quadriceps), ankles, and knees

Legs

- Stand with your feet shoulder-width apart
- Keep your heels flat, toes pointed straight ahead
- Assume a bent knee position (quarter squat)
- Hold 20–30 seconds

Stretches calves, Achilles area, and ankles; relaxes hamstrings

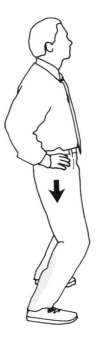

- Stand with your feet pointed straight ahead, a little more than shoulder-width apart
- Bend your left knee slightly and move your right hip downward toward your right knee
- Hold 10–15 seconds
- Repeat for the other leg

Stretches inner thighs and groin

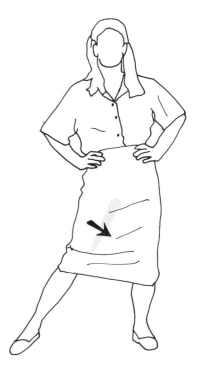

- Sitting, hold onto your upper left leg just above and behind the knee
- Gently pull your bent leg toward your chest
- Hold 10–15 seconds
- Repeat other side

Stretches hamstrings and lower back

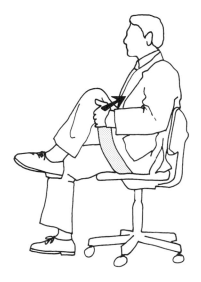

- Stand with hands on your hips
- Gently turn your torso at the waist and look over your shoulder until you feel the stretch
- Hold 8–10 seconds
- Repeat other side
- Keep your knees slightly flexed
- Do not hold your breath

Stretches back and sides

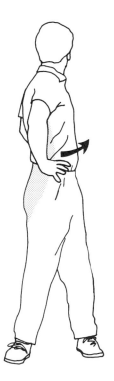

- Sit with your left leg bent over your right leg
- Rest the hand of your right arm on the outside of your upper left thigh
- Apply steady, controlled pressure toward the right with your hand
- As you do this, look over your left shoulder and feel the stretch
- Hold 5–10 seconds
- Repeat other side
- Breathe slowly

Stretches lower back, side of hip, and neck

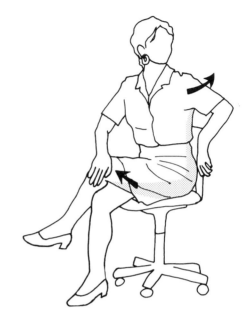

- Place your hands shoulder-width apart on a file cabinet or the wall
- Bend your knees; hips directly above feet
- Lower your head between your arms
- Hold stretch 10–15 seconds

Stretches neck, shoulders, arms, upper back

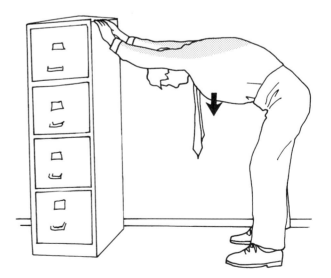

- Lean forward to stretch
- Keep your head down and your neck relaxed
- Hold 10–20 seconds
- Use your hands to push yourself upright

Stretches back

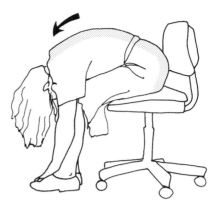

Face

- Raise your eyebrows and open your eyes wide
- At the same time, open your mouth to stretch your facial muscles
- Hold 5 seconds

Relaxes face, relieves jaw tension (and makes other people laugh!)

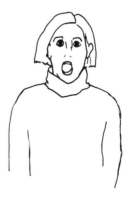

Office Exercises

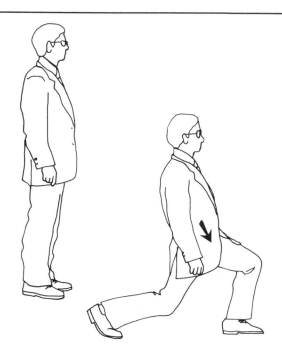

Front Lunge

- Head up, back straight, feet 6 inches apart
- Step forward as shown
- Return to standing position
- Try to keep back leg straight
- Repeat with other leg

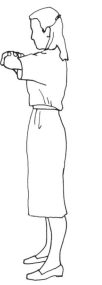
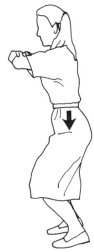

Quarter Squat

- Arms crossed in front of chest
- Head up, back straight, feet 16 inches apart
- Squat as shown
- Return to standing position

Chest Press

- Stand with hands against a door jamb
- Feet shoulder-width apart
- Lean forward, bending arms at elbows
- Press back to standing position

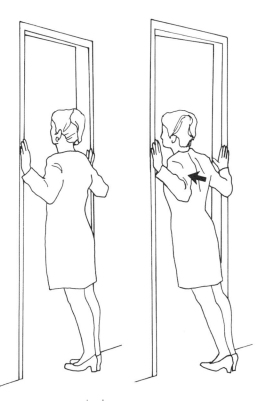

Toe Raise

- Stand about 40 inches from a door or the wall
- Lean forward, arms crossed
- Back straight, head up, legs locked
- Rise on toes as high as possible
- Come back down

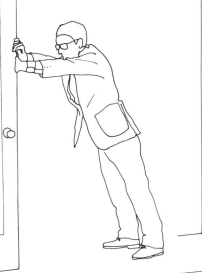

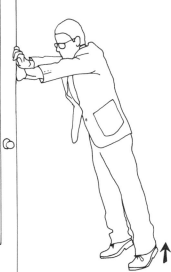

Office Exercises

Squat

- Holding onto doorknobs, stand straight, feet shoulder-width apart
- Bend knees and squat (only as far as is comfortable)
- Return to standing position
- Keep arms straight

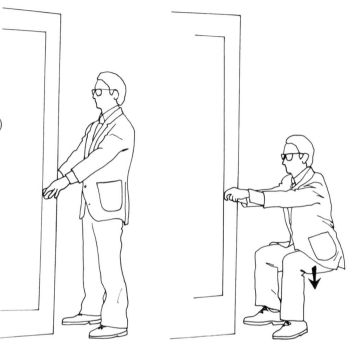

Desk Pushup

- Feet together, hand on desk at arm's length
- Inhale and press forward, bending arms at elbows
- Legs straight, heels down
- Return to standing position and exhale

It Couldn't Be Simpler

Remember: You can stretch anywhere, any time. Indoors or out, no special clothes needed. No classes to attend, no teacher required . . .

Appendix

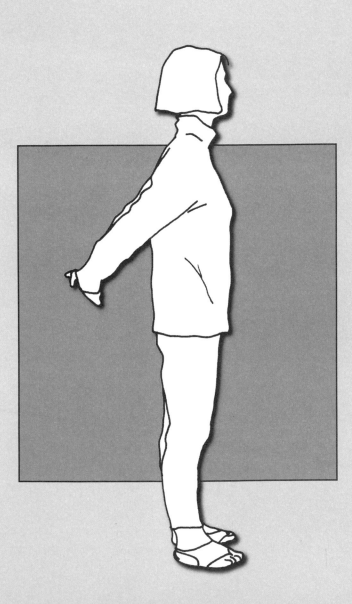

Bibliography

Rather than present a long list of reference material, we have selected the best books, newsletters, catalogs, and Web sites on the subject and reviewed them here for your convenience.

BOOKS ON ERGONOMICS

Compute in Comfort by Paul Linden (Prentice Hall PTR: Upper Saddle River, NY, 1995).

A practical book with exercises for preventing computer stress, tips on posture, proper sitting, healthy functioning of various body parts, and detailed descriptions of setting up a workstation. The author does not agree with many commonly accepted ergonomic principles and offers unique tips on adjusting and even building a workstation tailor-made to your needs. This is perhaps the best book out there on using the body in a stress-free and comfortable way and for customizing a workstation. There is a section on how to work with a drawing tablet, how to use a laptop, and setting up a standing workstation. A unique and detailed approach.

The Computer User's Survival Guide by Joan Stigliani (O'Reilly & Associates: Sebastapol, CA, 1995).

A comprehensive, user-friendly book on staying healthy while working at computers. The focus is on self-treatment; a chapter called "The Nature of the Beast" divides repetitive strain injuries into tendon injuries, muscle injuries, and nerve disorders, and there is good information on stress. Excellent index of resources, including product catalogs, newsletters, support groups, books, and research on electromagnetic fields.

25 Steps to Safe Computing by Don Sellers (Peachpit Press: Berkeley, CA, 1995).

A small, slim volume from the computer gurus at Peachpit Press. Information is in bite-sized bits, clear, and readily accessible. An excellent (and inexpensive) guide for employers to give to each employee to foster safe computing habits. It's simple, well researched, helpful, easy to understand, and particularly suited to today's busy lifestyle. Covers the basics on office health, how to keep the body functioning, safe workstations, finding the right doctor, and the subject of pregnancy and computing. Keep it in your desk.

Zap! How Your Computer Can Hurt You and What You Can Do About it by Don Sellers (Peachpit Press: Berkeley, CA, 1995).

Same author as preceding book. This is more comprehensive and detailed on computer-related injuries and remedies. Sellers states that over 4 million people in the United States suffer from some type of RSI and that over 60% of all workplace illnesses are RSIs. His approach is to minimize chances that your computer will hurt you and to provide info and exercises to prevent RSI's. Covers many subjects, including monitor radiation, ergonomic principles, lighting and air suggestions, back pain, carpal tunnel syndrome, etc. Very large, complete reference section, probably the best of any book.

Vision Comfort at VDTs – The Ergonomic Positioning of Monitors and Work Documents by Stewart B. Leavitt (MicroCentre, 5300 N. Irwindale Ave. Irwindale CA, 91706; 1-800-966-5511). Available free.

This is an excellent (if somewhat technical) 25-page pamphlet on eyestrain and video. Leavitt concludes that most people place their monitors too high for comfortable vision and that the height should be determined, not by the usual "top-of-monitor-at-eye-level" rule, but rather by visual acuity of the user, monitor size and quality, type of work performed, and size of type. While the thrust of the treatise is to recommend workstation setups, it has a very thorough and interesting discussion of human vision and what factors can cause discomfort or difficulty in using computers and reading paper documents.

BOOKS ON INJURIES

The Carpal Tunnel Syndrome Book by Mark A. Pinsky (Warner Books, New York, NY, 1993).

This is an inexpensive pocketbook with a slightly misleading title. It covers a range of cumulative trauma disorders, *including* carpal tunnel syndrome. If you have any RSI-type problem, it would be good to read this book so you know something about the subject when talking to a doctor. There are some self-administered screening techniques you can do to tell what type of problem you have. Interestingly, the author says the injuries may be far more prevalent than federal statistics indicate. Labor unions contend that there may be between 10 and 20 million people with cumulative trauma disorders!

Conquering Carpal Tunnel Syndrome by Sharon J. Butler (Advanced Press, Berwyn, PA, 1995).

Over 40 stretches and exercises for people with repetitive strain injuries. There is a cross-reference from the type problem (tingling fingers, painful elbows, etc.) to the exercises designed to alleviate the condition. There is also a chart of professions with recommended exercises for each group; one set of exercises for architects and dental hygenists, another set for carpenters and guitarists, etc. A unique feature is the number of stretches for wrists hands, fingers, and thumbs. The author practices Hellerwork, an offshoot of Rolfing, and stresses freeing up the body's connective tissue, or myofascia, to restore it to a more normal state, thereby regaining flexibility and range of motion.

Listen to Your Pain: The Active Person's Guide to Understanding, Identifying and Treating Pain and Injury by Ben E. Benjamin, Ph.D. (Penguin Books, New York, NY, 1984).

This is a book primarily for injured athletes, but it is also the best book available on injuries in general, whether they come from sports, accidents, or gradual wear and tear. (An exception is that it does not cover hand, wrist, or forearm problems.) It is divided up by body parts and gives you unique methods for self-diagnosis to identify what the injury is, followed with step-by-step remedies to facilitate healing. An excellent reference book for the home library.

Repetitive Strain Injury by Emil Pascarelli, M.D., and Deborah Quilter (John Wiley & Sons, New York, NY, 1994).

One of the best books on RSI, written by a doctor with a great deal of experience—he has worked with over 1,000 injured people, many of them musicians. He calls RSI "a preventable tragedy," describes the warning signs, classifies different types of RSI (the latter is particularly concise and informative), explains treatment options, and talks about setting up the workstation. There is a good section called "The Road to Recovery," with advice on dealing with a doctor, self care, working during the recovery phase, activities of daily living, and preventing further injuries.

Soft Tissue Pain and Disability by Rene Cailliet, M.D. (F. A. Davis, Philadelphia, PA, 1977).

Rene Cailliet has written a well-regarded series of books covering injuries to various parts of the body. These are intended more for doctors than lay persons, but include common-sense guidance for diagnosis and treatment that may be useful to patients wishing to discuss their symptoms in depth with their doctors. This volume covers soft-tissue injuries of the low back, neck, arm, shoulder, elbow, wrist, hand, hip, knee, foot, and ankle. Clear drawings.

Bibliography

BOOKS ON GENERAL FITNESS

Stretching by Bob Anderson; illustrated by Jean Anderson (Shelter Publications, Bolinas, CA, 1980).

One of the most popular fitness books in the world, with over 2 million copies sold and translated into 16 languages. A clear, readable, graphic summary of 200 different stretches with 1- and 2-page routines for everyday stretches, TV stretches, stretches for lower back pain, to do after sitting, before walking, as well as stretching programs for over 20 sports. There is a "Stretching & Exercise Prescriptions" index in the back of the book that can be used by readers or medical professionals to design customized stretching programs.

Getting in Shape by Bob Anderson, Bill Pearl and Ed Burke; illustrated by Jean Anderson (Shelter Publications, Bolinas, CA, 1994).

A unique and comprehensive workout book for people who want to get back into shape. The authors feel that most fitness books are too ambitious for the average person and have produced a book that can be tailor-made to each person's individual condition. There is a series of graphic programs starting with the 3-stage "Program Before the Program" designed to get you started when you're out of shape. There are 30 programs overall, each with the 3 components of fitness: stretching, weightlifting, and moving exercise. A simple, easy to follow, and visual approach to lifetime fitness, especially useful for the over-40 adult.

Living with Exercise: Improving Your Health Through Moderate Physical Activity by Steven N. Blair, P.E.D. (American Health Publishing Company, Dallas TX, 1991).

A very important fitness book—for the average American. This is no hardcore, high-achievement, high-performance approach to fitness, but rather a more gentle, easy-going guide. "Doing something is better than doing nothing," says Blair and he shows you how to work increased activity into your daily routine and include exercise as part of a busy schedule. This book marked a change in attitude on the American fitness scene and the message is encouraging and inspiring. Says Blair, "Exercise needn't hurt. . . ."

RSI NEWSLETTERS

CTD News
P.O. Box 980, Horsham, PA 19044-0980
(800-341-7874)
http://ctdnews.com/

Monthly newsletter aimed at businesses concerned with repetitive strain injuries or cumulative trauma disorders and giving up-to-date news on ergonomic safety. For example, a recent issue covered the relatively new use of angioplasty in CTS to stretch wrist and hand ligaments, thereby bypassing the need for surgery. Free samples of newsletter sent upon request.

RSI Newsletter
http://www.safecomputing.com/

Available only on the Web, this is a newsletter of interest to people who have repetetive strain injuries. Information on ergonomic safety.

ERGONOMIC CATALOGS

AliMed Ergonomic Products
P.O. Box 9135, Dedham, MA, 02027-9135
(800-225-2610)

Large catalog of wrist straps, many other ergonomic office products, mainly for professionals. They publish a shorter magazine called *Ergonomics and Occupational Health.*

Fellowes Computerware.
1789 Norwood Ave., Itasca, IL, 60143
(800-945-4545)

Fellowes manufactures over 400 computer accessory products—wrist rests, monitor filters, seating supports, copy stands, adjustable monitor arms, cordless mouse pens, etc., many of them original design. They have an ergonomic task force that specializes in working with corporations interested in safe ergonomic practices. A complete list of products available upon request.

The North American Ergonomic Resources Guide
Published by CTD News,
P.O. Box 980, Horsham, PA 19044-0980
(800-341-7874)

This is an excellent compendium of information on all aspects of ergonomics: a listing of many catalogs of ergonomic products and furniture; alternative keyboards and mice, voice control systems, books, videos, software, other resources. There are also nationwide lists of ergonomic consultants, educational conferences, and databases.

Saunders Ergosource
4250 Noprex Dr., Chaska MN 55318-3047
(800-969-4374)

Catalog of ergonomic aids, tools, furniture, and educational literature.

Upper Extremity Technology Products
UE Tech, 2001 Blake Ave., 2-A,
Glenwood Springs, CO 81601
(800-736-1894)

Catalog contains a number of books on repetitive motion injuries, ergonomic design, rehabilitation, etc. "By therapists . . . for therapists."

WORLDWIDE WEB

Computer-related Repetitive Strain Injury
http://engr-www.unl.edu/ee/eeshop/rsi.html

This is an excellent site for sound ergonomic principles and the basics of RSI without being boring or academic. Webmaster Paul Marxhausen has had RSI problems since 1994 and urges people with any of the listed symptoms to ". . . run, do not walk, to your doctor or health care provider *right away.*" He is aware of the value of early diagnosis and treatment. There are links to other sites, products, and resources, including "FindADoc," aimed at locating doctors specializing in RSI throughout the country.

Typing Injury FAQ: A Guide to Comfortable Computing.
http://www.cs.princeton.edu/~dwallach/tifaq/

This is the granddaddy of online RSI information sites. Tons of information here, with links going off in many directions to all kinds of data on the subject. Lots of info on products such as keyboards, alternative pointing devices, desks and chairs, a very complete list of various software programs that will remind you to stretch while at the keyboard, and an archive of typing injuries.

Shelter Online
http://www.shelterpub.com

Shelter Publications' website, with information on stretching, (including—ahem!—programs from this book), weight training, running, fitness in general, healthy cooking, and a variety of other subjects.

INTERNET NEWSGROUPS

Sorehand

A very active newsgroup of people with computer-related problems. These are the people in the trenches. If you subscribe, be forewarned, you will get a ton of e-mail. Much of it is helpful and up-to-date—an example of the unique facility of Internet information exchange. The irony is that the helpful data comes to you through the same device that is causing the trouble.

To subscribe, send message "subscribe sorehand <your name>" to: listserv@itssrvl.ucsf.edu

C+health

Another excellent source of info on RSI, with contributors from around the world. There's something unique and especially relevant about these personal accounts from many people with the same problems. The network of people helping one another is useful as well as inspiring, and the exchanges are more current than is available in any other media.

To subscribe, send message "subscribe c+health <your name>" to: listserv@iubvm.ucs.indiana.edu

Body Tools

Sometimes you need a helping hand—or a helping tool—to make you feel better. Listed on these 2 pages are body tools that can be used for self-massage and loosening up in the office. They help relieve pain and tension. All but The Back Revolution® can be kept in or on your desk.

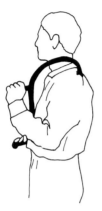

TheraCane®: acupressure tool. Loosens tight, painful areas— creates the pressure you want. Excellent for mid-back (between shoulder blades), sides of neck, shoulders.

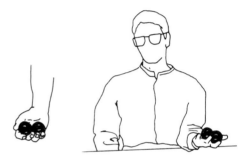

Chinese Balls: exercise for your hands. Rotating balls in one direction, then another develops small muscles of hands, improves arm circulation, may help prevent carpal tunnel syndrome.

Trigger Wheel®: 2-inch nylon wheel on 4½-inch handle for deep massage. Works on trigger points of muscles. Can use directly on skin or through light clothing. It works the way a tire rolls back and forth on the pavement.

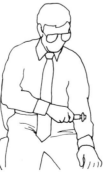

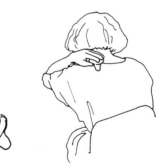

Knobble®: small hand tool for doing deep tissue massage or pressure point release. Saves wear and tear on your hands. Made of solid maple.

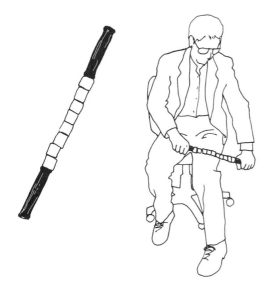

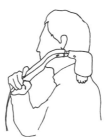

Panasonic Shiatsu Accutap II®: tapping massage stimulates muscles, relieves tension. Especially good for neck and shoulder stiffness. Two levels of intensity, 10 speeds. Keep it by your computer. (When you are using just the mouse with one hand, you can use this device to loosen up your neck and shoulders with the other hand.)

The Stick®: non-motorized massage device. Used by serious athletes to loosen "barrier trigger points" (knotted-up muscles). Flexible core has revolving spindles.

See p. 99 for information on ordering any of these tools.

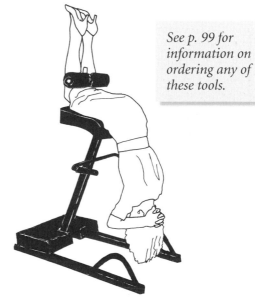

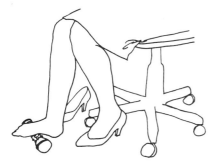

The Foot Massage®: 2 inches by 9 inches, with raised knobs of hard rubber for foot massage and rubber rings to protect floors. Super tool for tired feet.

The Back Revolution®: Truly a revolution, much better than hanging by heels, this stretches spine, decompresses discs and works wonders for sore, stiff necks. Benefits accrue from using it only 1 to 2 times daily.

Index of Stretches

Here are all the stretches in the book. This allows you to select stretches by body part. It can also serve as a guide for health care professionals in prescribing individual fitness or rehabilitation programs. Make a copy of this and circle the prescribed stretches.

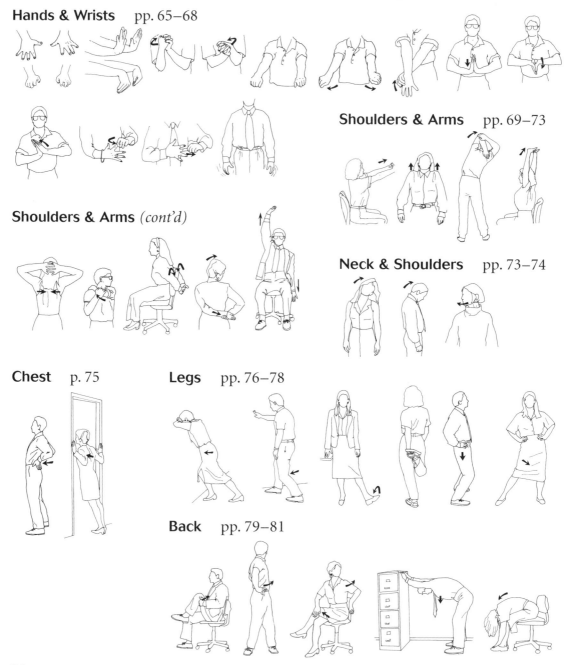

Hands & Wrists   pp. 65–68

Shoulders & Arms   pp. 69–73

Shoulders & Arms *(cont'd)*

Neck & Shoulders   pp. 73–74

Chest   p. 75

Legs   pp. 76–78

Back   pp. 79–81

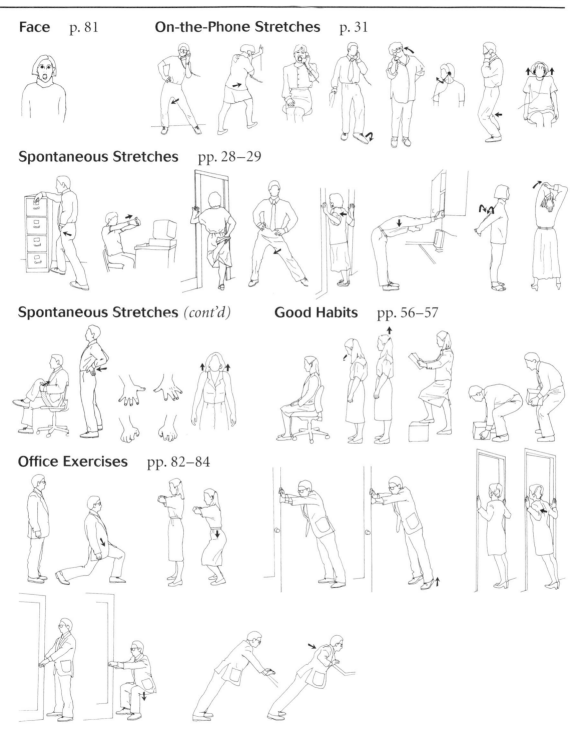

Face   p. 81

On-the-Phone Stretches   p. 31

Spontaneous Stretches   pp. 28–29

Spontaneous Stretches *(cont'd)*

Good Habits   pp. 56–57

Office Exercises   pp. 82–84

Stretching at Your Computer or Desk © 1997 Robert A. Anderson, Jean E. Anderson & Shelter Publications, Inc.

Index

Note: Page numbers in italics refer to illustrations.

About the Authors

Bob Anderson is the author of *Stretching,* which has sold over 2 million copies worldwide and is in 17 languages.* Bob was born in Fullerton, California, and is a graduate of California State University at Long Beach with a lifetime credential in physical education. These days, Bob travels around the country, appearing at medical clinics, health conventions, training camps, and fitness centers. His appearances generally involve getting (himself and audience) down on the floor and doing a series of gentle stretches. All the while Bob talks about good health and the importance of keeping one's body strong and flexible and keeping the heart and cardiovascular system in good shape.

Bob is fit and healthy these days, but it wasn't always so. In 1968, he was overweight (190 pounds—at 5 feet 9 inches) and out of shape. He began a personal fitness program that got him down to 135 pounds. Yet one day, while in a physical conditioning class in college, he found he couldn't reach much past his knees in a straight-legged sitting position. So Bob started stretching. He found he soon felt better and that stretching made his running and cycling easier.

Since that time, Bob has continued to practice what he preaches. He spends several hours each day running on the steep mountain trails above his house in Colorado and riding his mountain bike. He has run the Catalina Island Marathon in Southern California, the Pikes Peak Marathon 10 years in a row, and regularly runs the 18-mile Imogen Pass Run, a mountain race from Ouray to Telluride, Colorado, which goes up over a 13,000-foot-high ridge.

Though Bob works out long and hard each day, he knows that training like this is not for the average person. Through his travels, lectures, and workshops, he's kept in constant touch with people in all degrees of physical condition.

Jean Anderson, Bob's wife, plays a major role in the design and development of Stretching Inc.'s large line of stretching products *(see adjacent page).* Jean was born in Long Beach, California, and is a graduate of California State University at Long Beach, where she received her B.A. in art. In the early 70s, when Bob was teaching stretching to the Denver Broncos, the Los Angeles Lakers, and the New York Jets, Jean developed a system of doing line drawings from photos of Bob doing the stretches. Jean also works with Bob in developing the stretching instructions and creating and producing their various stretching books, posters, and videotapes.

*including Chinese, Lithuanian and Finnish

More on Stretching

From Bob and Jean Anderson

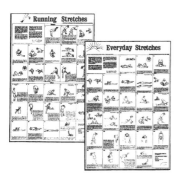

Stretching Posters

Easy-to-read, 22½ × 34 inch and 17 × 22 inch wall posters are great visual aids for learning how to stretch. A total of 48 posters on 35 different sports, on body parts (lower back, neck/shoulder/arms, groin and hip, etc.), and miscellaneous subjects such as pregnancy, over 50, kids' stretches, partner stretches. Also a wall chart on computer and desk stretches that can be posted in the office. All posters available in laminated versions.

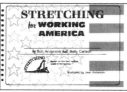

Stretching for Working America by Bob Anderson and Sally Carlson

Written for workers, people who work with their hands and bodies. Stretching before doing physical labor has been proven to reduce workplace injuries. The programs can be used by the individual worker or as part of an organized program for business, large or small.

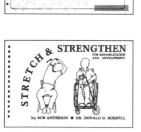

Stretch and Strengthen by Bob Anderson and Dr. Donald G. Bornell

Individual stretching and strengthening exercises instruct people in wheelchairs, the disabled, and elderly. Also an excellent tool for rehabilitation. Comes with "Isoband" elastic exercise band for progressive resistance training to be done while sitting.

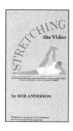

Stretching, The Video

A 57-minute video that is organized into comfortably paced sections. First there is an introduction to stretching. Then body parts, divided into neck and back, then legs and hips, followed by stretches for the feet and then arms and shoulders. Then there is a 14-minute program to use for everyday fitness or for specific sports and activities.

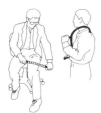

Body Tools

Excellent aids in helping reduce muscle tension and pain. All of these can be used in the office. *(See pp. 92 to 93.)*

To contact Stretching, Inc. *for a free 4-color catalog of these and other fitness products, write Stretching, Inc., P.O. Box 767, Palmer Lake, CO, 80133 or call 800-333-1307.*

E-mail: *stretch@usa.net*   **Website:** *http://www.stretching.com*

Fax–a–Friend

Photocopy and fax one or two of the routines in this book to a friend you think might benefit from stretching. You can use this page as a cover letter.

✂ cut photocopy here

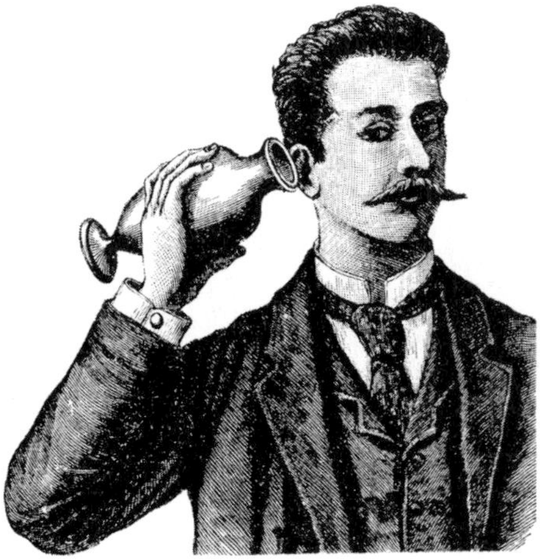

FAX

Date _____

To _____

Fax # _____

This cover sheet followed by _____ pages

Message: _____

_____

_____

_____

_____

_____

_____

From: _____

_____

Credits

Editor
Lloyd Kahn

Contributing Editors
Stuart Kenter
George Young

Art Director
David Wills

Design
Rick Gordon
Lloyd Kahn

Design Consultant
Janet Bollow

Cover Design
David Wills

Production Manager
Rick Gordon

Production Assistant
Christina Reski

Proofreading & Indexing
Frances Bowles

Models for Drawings
Bob Anderson
Jean Anderson
Joan Creed
Linda Donahue
Bob Kahn
Kay Labella
Grace London
Christina Reski
Dave Roche
Vandy Seeburg
JoAnne Sercl
Peggy Sterling
Sandy Thomas
Joyce Werth

Special thanks to the following people, who helped with this book in one way or another:
Sally Carlson
Joan Creed
Page Dickinson
Michelle Donahue
Lesley Kahn
Paul Marxhausen
Maureen Watts

Production Hardware
Macintosh Quadra 950 64MB/2GB
Agfa Arcus II Scanner
Laserwriter Pro 600

Production Software
QuarkXpress® 3.31
Adobe Photoshop® 3.0.5
Adobe Illustrator® 6.0

Typefaces
Adobe Minion, Cosmos,
Zapf Dingbats

Paper
70# Bookmaster Matte

Binding
RepKover lay-flat binding with
cloth-reinforced backing

Printing
Courier Companies, Inc., Westford, MA

The World's Best Fitness Books

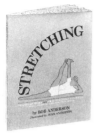

Stretching by Bob Anderson, illustrated by Jean Anderson © 1980; 192 pages, paperback; ISBN 0-394-73874-8
$13.00

A classic (2 million copies, in 17 languages). If you enjoy the stretching in *Stretching at Your Computer or Desk,* this book covers the subject in detail. Routines for 24 sports, and stretches to do when you get up in the morning, while watching TV, for everyday, for those over 50, etc.

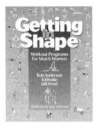

Getting in Shape by Bob Anderson, Bill Pearl and Ed Burke © 1994; 220 pages, paperback; ISBN 0-679-75609-4
$15.00

The best all-around fitness book in the world. Contains 30 programs, each with the three components of fitness: stretching, weight training, and moving exercises. You can choose your own level of commitment. For people who want to get back in shape, and for those who need to fit exercise into a busy schedule.

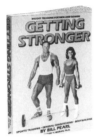

Getting Stronger by Bill Pearl and Gary T. Moran, Ph.D. © 1986; 464 pages, paperback; ISBN 0-679-73269-1
$19.00

The most popular weight training book in America, this is actually three books in one: general conditioning, sports training, and bodybuilding. Over 350 exercises for free weights, Nautilus, and the new electronic resistance machines. Bill Pearl is a four-time Mr. Universe.

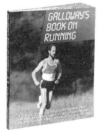

Galloway's Book on Running by Jeff Galloway © 1984; 288 pages, paperback; ISBN 0-394-72709-6
$13.00

Olympic runner Jeff Galloway shows how the same principles used by elite runners apply to runners of all levels. Jeff shows beginners how to get started, how to stay motivated, how to make running an integral part of one's life. There are training programs for 10K races and marathons. The best-selling running book in America.

All books available at your favorite bookstore
Distributed by Random House, Inc.

To order by mail, send price of book + $3.00 postage and handling to Shelter Publications, Inc. P.O. Box 279, Bolinas, CA, 94924, USA. • Phone: 415-868-0280 • E-mail: shelter@shelterpub.com. To order online, visit our Website. Or write or e-mail for for free catalog.

Visit us on the Web — http://www.shelterpub.com